P9-EFJ-049

"*The Upside of Stress* delivers an important truth: It is better to chase meaning than try to avoid discomfort. Through the insights of this book, you'll find your courage to pursue what matters most and trust yourself to handle any stress that follows."

—NILOFER MERCHANT, founder and CEO of
Rubicon Consulting, Silicon Valley
strategist, and author of *The New How*

"Kelly McGonigal has pulled back the curtain to reveal what allows exceptional people and organizations like my Navy SEAL brotherhood to thrive through adversity. True excellence is only achieved under great adversity and by embracing those challenges with a positive mindset."

—SCOTT BRAUER, cofounder of Acumen Performance
Group and former Navy SEAL and U.S. Navy officer

"The upside of Kelly McGonigal is that she not only shows how what we thought we knew about stress was backward, but also that getting it right will change your life for the better. This book provides an accessible user's guide to leveraging the most cutting-edge research in psychology and neuroscience to enhance your health and well-being."

—MATTHEW D. LIEBERMAN, PhD, chair of Social
Psychology at University of California, Los Angeles

"For those individuals and teams that discover stress *is* life's secret ingredient, they will be rewarded with expanded self-confidence and rapidly growing organizations."

—ROBERT C. DAUGHERTY, chairman of Knowledge
Investment Partners

"Kelly McGonigal debunks decades of myths that have persisted around stress. *The Upside of Stress* is research based, immensely practical, compelling, and insightful from the first page. This book will be a game changer for countless people."

—JIM LOEHR, EdD, cofounder of the Human
Performance Institute and author of
The New Toughness Training for Sports

PRAISE FOR *THE WILLPOWER INSTINCT*

"Tired of the endless debate about whether man possesses free will or is predestined to lounge about gobbling Krispy Kreme donuts while watching TV? If you want action, not theory, *The Willpower Instinct* is the solution for the chronically slothful."

—*USA Today*

"A fun and readable survey of the field, bringing willpower wisdom out of the labs."

—*Time* magazine

"Refreshingly easy to read and peppered with stories of people who have successfully used its methods, *The Willpower Instinct* is a new kind of self-help book. Using science to help explain the 'why,' and strategies for the 'how,' McGonigal has created a book that will appeal to those who want to lose a few pounds as well as those who are eager to understand why they just cannot seem to get through their to-do list. A must-read for anyone who wants to change how they live in both small and big ways."

—*BookPage*

"*The Willpower Instinct* combines the braininess of a Malcolm Gladwell bestseller with the actual helpfulness of an Idiots' Guide to not being lazy. If you are trying to lose weight, train for an athletic event, become more successful at work, rid yourself of toxic habits . . . heck, if you're human, you need to read this book."

—*LibraryThing*

"This book has tremendous value for anyone interested in learning how to achieve their goals more effectively. McGonigal clearly breaks down a large body of relevant scientific research and its applications, and shows that awareness of the limits of willpower is crucial to our ability to exercise true self-control."

—JEFFREY M. SCHWARTZ, MD, author of the bestselling *Brain Lock*

"What a liberating book! Kelly McGonigal explains the scientific reality of willpower, exploding the myths that most of us believe. Stronger willpower—based on inspiring facts, not oppressive nonsense—is finally within everyone's reach."

—GEOFF COLVIN, author of *Talent Is Overrated*

The Upside *of* STRESS

The Upside of STRESS

why stress is good for you, and how to get good at it

Kelly McGonigal, Ph.D.

AVERY
a member of Penguin Random House
New York

AVERY

An imprint of Penguin Random House
375 Hudson Street
New York, New York 10014

Most Avery books are available at special quantity discounts for bulk purchase for sales promotions,
premiums, fund-raising, and educational needs. Special books or book excerpts also can
be created to fit specific needs. For details, write SpecialMarkets@penguinrandomhouse.com.

ISBN: 978-1-58333-561-1 (hardcover edition)
ISBN: 978-1-58333-589-5 (international edition)

Printed in the United States of America
1   3   5   7   9   10   8   6   4   2

Book design by Tanya Maiboroda

PUBLISHER'S NOTE

Neither the publisher nor the author is engaged in rendering professional advice or services to the individual reader. The ideas, procedures, and suggestions contained in this book are not intended as a substitute for consulting with your physician. All matters regarding your health require medical supervision. Neither the author nor the publisher shall be liable or responsible for any loss or damage allegedly arising from any information or suggestion in this book.

While the author has made every effort to provide accurate telephone numbers, Internet addresses, and other contact information at the time of publication, neither the publisher nor the author assumes any responsibility for errors, or for changes that occur after publication. Further, the publisher does not have any control over and does not assume any responsibility for author or third-party websites or their content.

AUTHOR'S NOTE

Throughout the book, when only first names are used, the names are pseudonyms, and some details of the stories have been changed to protect individuals' privacy. Whenever possible, I obtained permission to use these stories. If direct quotes are included in the stories, they are from email or personal exchanges and have not been altered. In all other cases, where full names are used, all quotes and details are from interviews I conducted and/or from published sources cited in the notes.

"If you have butterflies in your stomach,
invite them into your heart."

—COOPER EDENS

contents

introduction

I F YOU HAD to sum up how you feel about stress, which statement would be more accurate?"

A) Stress is harmful and should be avoided, reduced, and managed.
B) Stress is helpful and should be accepted, utilized, and embraced.

Five years ago, I would have chosen A without a moment's hesitation. I'm a health psychologist, and through all my training in psychology and medicine, I got one message loud and clear: Stress is toxic.

For years, as I taught classes and workshops, conducted research, and wrote articles and books, I took that message and ran with it. I told people that stress makes you sick; that it increases your risk of everything from the common cold to heart disease, depression, and addiction; and that it kills brain cells, damages your DNA, and makes you age faster. In media outlets ranging from the *Washington Post* to *Martha Stewart Weddings*, I gave the kind of stress-reduction advice you've probably heard a thousand times. Practice deep breathing, get more sleep, manage your time. And, of course, do whatever you can to reduce the stress in your life.

I turned stress into the enemy, and I wasn't alone. I was just one of many psychologists, doctors, and scientists crusading against stress. Like them, I believed that it was a dangerous epidemic that had to be stopped.

But I've changed my mind about stress, and now I want to change yours.

Let me start by telling you about the shocking scientific finding that first made me rethink stress. In 1998, thirty thousand adults in the United States were asked how much stress they had experienced in the past year. They were also asked, Do you believe stress is harmful to your health?

Eight years later, the researchers scoured public records to find out who among the thirty thousand participants had died. Let me deliver the bad news first. High levels of stress increased the risk of dying by 43 percent. But—and this is what got my attention—that increased risk applied only to people who also believed that stress was harming their health. People who reported high levels of stress but who did not view their stress as harmful were not more likely to die. In fact, they had the lowest risk of death of anyone in the study, even lower than those who reported experiencing very little stress.

The researchers concluded that it wasn't stress alone that was killing people. It was the combination of stress and the *belief* that stress is harmful. The researchers estimated that over the eight years they conducted their study, 182,000 Americans may have died prematurely because they believed that stress was harming their health.

That number stopped me in my tracks. We're talking over twenty thousand deaths a year! According to statistics from the Centers for Disease Control and Prevention, that would make "believing stress is bad for you" the fifteenth-leading cause of death in the United States, killing more people than skin cancer, HIV/AIDS, and homicide.

As you can imagine, this finding unnerved me. Here I was, spending all this time and energy convincing people that stress was bad for their health. I had completely taken for granted that this message—and my work—was helping people. But what if it wasn't? Even if the techniques I was teaching for stress reduction—such as physical exercise, meditation, and social connection—were truly helpful, was I undermining their benefit by delivering them alongside the message that stress is toxic? Was it possible that in the name of stress management, I had been doing more harm than good?

I admit, I was tempted to pretend that I never saw that study. After all, it was just one study—and a correlational study at that! The researchers had looked at a wide range of factors that might explain the finding, including gender, race, ethnicity, age, education, income, work status, marital status, smoking, physical activity, chronic health condition, and health insurance. None of these things explained why stress beliefs interacted with stress levels to predict mortality. However, the researchers hadn't actually manipulated people's beliefs about stress, so they couldn't be sure that it *was* people's beliefs that were killing them. Was it possible that people who believe that their stress is harmful have a different kind of stress in their lives—one that is, somehow, more toxic? Or perhaps they have personalities that make them particularly vulnerable to the harmful effects of stress.

And yet, I couldn't get the study out of my head. In the midst of my self-doubt, I also sensed an opportunity. I'd always told my psychology students at Stanford University that the most exciting kind of scientific finding is one that challenges how you think about yourself and the world. But then I found the tables were turned. Was I ready to have my own beliefs challenged?

The finding I had stumbled across—that stress is harmful only when you believe it is—offered me an opportunity to rethink what I was teaching. Even more, it was an invitation to rethink my own relationship to stress. Would I seize it? Or would I file away the paper and continue to crusade against stress?

Two things in my training as a health psychologist made me open to the idea that how you think about stress matters—and to the possibility that telling people "Stress will kill you!" could have unintended consequences.

First, I was already aware that some beliefs can influence longevity. For example, people with a positive attitude about aging live longer than those who hold negative stereotypes about getting older. One classic study by researchers at Yale University followed middle-aged adults for twenty years. Those who had a positive view of aging in midlife lived an average of 7.6 years longer than those who had a negative view. To put that number in perspective, consider this: Many things we regard as obvious and important protective factors, such as exercising regularly, not smoking, and maintaining healthy blood pressure and cholesterol levels, have been shown, on average, to add less than four years to one's life span.

Another example of a belief with long-reaching impact has to do with trust. Those who believe that most people can be trusted tend to live longer. In a fifteen-year study by Duke University researchers, 60 percent of adults over the age of fifty-five who viewed others as trustworthy were still alive at the end of the study. In contrast, 60 percent of those with a more cynical view on human nature had died.

Findings like these had already convinced me that when it comes to health and longevity, some beliefs matter. But what I didn't know yet was whether how you think about stress was one of them.

The second thing that made me willing to admit I might be wrong about stress was what I know about the history of health promotion. If telling people that stress is killing them is a bad strategy for public health, it wouldn't be the first time a popular health promotion strategy backfired. Some of the most commonly used strategies to encourage healthy behavior have been found to do exactly the opposite of what health professionals hope.

For example, when I speak with physicians, I sometimes ask them to predict the effects of showing smokers graphic warnings on cigarette packs. In general, they believe that the images will decrease smokers' desire for a cigarette and motivate them to quit. But studies show that the warnings often have the reverse effect. The most threatening images (say, a lung cancer patient dying in a hospital bed) actually *increase* smokers' positive attitudes toward smoking. The reason? The images trigger fear, and what better way to calm down than to smoke a cigarette? The doctors assumed that the fear would inspire behavior change, but instead it just motivates a desire to escape feeling bad.

Another strategy that consistently backfires is shaming people for their unhealthy behaviors. In one study at the University of California, Santa Barbara, overweight women read a *New York Times* article about how employers are beginning to discriminate against overweight workers. Afterward, instead of vowing to lose weight, the women ate twice as many calories of junk food as overweight women who had read an article on a different workplace issue.

Fear, stigma, self-criticism, shame—all of these are believed, by many health professionals, to be powerfully motivating messages that help people improve their well-being. And yet, when put to the scientific test, these messages push people toward the very behaviors the health professionals hope to change. Over the years, I've seen the same dynamic play out: Well-intentioned doctors and psychologists convey a message they think will help; instead, the recipients end up overwhelmed, depressed, and driven to self-destructive coping behaviors.

After I first discovered the study linking beliefs about stress to mortality, I started to pay more attention to how people reacted when

I talked about the harmful effects of stress. I noticed that my message was met with the same kind of overwhelming feeling I would expect from medical warnings intended to frighten or shame. When I told exhausted undergraduate students about the negative consequences of stress right before final exam period, the students left the lecture hall more depressed. When I shared scary statistics about stress with caregivers, sometimes there were tears. No matter the audience, nobody ever came up afterward to say, "Thank you so much for telling me how toxic my stressful life is. I know I can get rid of the stress, but I'd just never thought to do it before!"

I realized that as much as I believed talking about stress was important, how I was doing it might not be helping. Everything I had been taught about stress management started from the assumption that stress is dangerous and that people needed to know this. Once they understood how bad stress was, they would reduce their stress, and this would make them healthier and happier. But now, I wasn't so sure.

MY CURIOSITY about how your attitude toward stress influences its impact sent me on a search for more evidence. I wanted to know: Does how you think about stress really matter? And if believing that stress is bad *is* bad for you, what's the alternative? Is there anything good about stress that's worth embracing?

As I pored over scientific studies and surveys from the past three decades, I looked at the data with an open mind. I found evidence for some of the harmful effects we fear but also for benefits we rarely recognize. I investigated the history of stress, learning more about how psychology and medicine became convinced that it is toxic. I also talked to scientists who are part of a new generation of stress researchers, whose work is redefining our understanding of stress by illuminating its upside. What I learned from these studies, surveys, and conversations truly changed the way I think about stress. The latest science reveals that stress can make you smarter, stronger, and more successful. It helps you learn and grow. It can even inspire courage and compassion.

The new science also shows that changing your mind about stress can make you healthier and happier. How you think about stress affects everything from your cardiovascular health to your ability to find meaning in life. The best way to manage stress isn't to reduce or avoid it, but rather to rethink and even embrace it.

So, my goal as a health psychologist has changed. I no longer want to help you get rid of your stress—I want to make you better at stress. That is the promise of the new science of stress, and the purpose of this book.

About This Book

This book is based on a course I teach through Stanford Continuing Studies called the New Science of Stress. The course, which enrolls people of all ages and from all walks of life, is designed to transform the way we think about and live with stress.

It's helpful to know a little about the science behind embracing stress for two reasons. First, it's fascinating. When the subject is human nature, every study is an opportunity to better understand yourself and those you care about. Second, the science of stress has some real surprises. Certain ideas about stress—including the central premise of this book: that stress can be good for you—are hard to swallow. Without evidence, it would be easy to dismiss them. Seeing the science behind these ideas can help you consider them and how they might apply to your own experiences.

The advice in this book isn't based on one shocking study—even though that's what inspired me to rethink stress. The strategies you'll learn are based on hundreds of studies and the insights of dozens of scientists I've spoken with. Skipping the science and getting straight to the advice doesn't work. Knowing what's behind every strategy helps them stick. So this book includes a crash course in the new science of stress and what psychologists call *mindsets*. You'll be introduced to rising-star researchers and some of their most intriguing studies—all in a way that I hope any reader can enjoy. If you have a bigger appetite for scientific details and want even more information, the notes at the end of this book will let you dig deeper.

But most important, this is a practical guide to getting better at living with stress. Embracing stress can make you feel more empowered in the face of challenges. It can enable you to better use the energy of stress without burning out. It can help you turn stressful experiences into a source of social connection rather than isolation. And finally, it can lead you to new ways of finding meaning in suffering.

Throughout this book, you'll find two types of practical exercises to try:

The Rethink Stress exercises in Part 1 are designed to shift your way of thinking about stress. You can use them as writing prompts or as any other forms of self-reflection that work for you. You might think about the topic while you're on the treadmill at the gym or riding the bus to work. You can make it a private reflection or use it to start a conversation. Talk about it with your spouse over dinner or bring it up at your parents' group at church. Write a Facebook post about it and ask your friends for their thoughts. Along with helping you think differently about stress in general, these exercises also encourage you to reflect on the role that stress plays in your life, including in relation to your most important goals and values.

The Transform Stress exercises in Part 2 include on-the-spot strategies to use in moments of stress, as well as self-reflections that will help you cope with specific challenges in your life. They will help you tap into your reserves of energy, strength, and hope when you're feeling anxious, frustrated, angry, or overwhelmed. Transform Stress exercises rely on what I call "mindset resets"—shifts in how you think about the stress you are experiencing in the moment. These mindset resets can alter your physical stress response, change your attitude, and motivate action. In other words, they transform the effect that stress is having on you in the very moment you are feeling stressed. These exercises are based on scientific studies, and I encourage you to treat them like experiments yourself. Try them out and see what works for you.

All the exercises in this book have been shaped by the feedback of my students and by my experiences sharing these ideas with communities around the world, including with educators, medical professionals, executives, professional coaches, family therapists, and parents. I've included the practices that people tell me have been personally and professionally meaningful, leading to change in their own lives and in the communities they work with.

Together, these exercises will help you change your relationship with stress. It might feel weird to think about having a relationship with stress, especially if you're used to thinking of stress as something that happens *to* you. But you do have a relationship with stress. You might feel victimized by stress—helpless against it or held hostage by it. Or maybe yours is a love-hate relationship—relying on stress to reach your goals but worried about its long-term consequences. Perhaps you feel like you are in a constant struggle with stress, trying to reduce, avoid, or manage it without ever being able to control it. Or maybe you feel like the stressful experiences in your past have too much sway over your present self. You might view stress as your enemy, an unwanted guest, or a partner you aren't quite sure you can trust. Whatever your current relationship with stress, how you think about it and how you respond to it both play an important role in how it affects you. By rethinking and even embracing stress, you can change its effect on everything from your physical health and emotional well-being to your satisfaction at work and hopefulness about the future.

Throughout the book, we'll also consider how the science of stress and mindsets can help you support the people, communities, and organizations you care about. How can we nurture resilience in our loved ones? What would it look like for a workplace culture to embrace stress? How do people build support networks to deal with trauma or loss? I'll introduce you to some of my favorite programs that are using this science to create communities that are able to transform suffering into growth, meaning, and connection. These programs can serve as models and inspiration, demonstrating what it looks like to translate science into service, and abstract ideas into actions with impact.

Will This Book Help Me with My Stress?

So far, I've avoided defining *stress*—in part because the word has become a catchall term for anything we don't want to experience and everything that's wrong with the world. People use the word *stress* to describe both a traffic delay and a death in the family. We say we're stressed when we feel anxious, busy, frustrated, threatened, or under pressure. On any given day, you might find yourself getting stressed out by email, politics, the news, the weather, or your growing to-do list. And the biggest source of stress in your life right now could be work, parenting, dealing with a health crisis, getting out of debt, or going through a divorce. Sometimes we use the word *stress* to describe what's going on inside us—our thoughts, emotions, and physical responses—and sometimes we use it describe the problems we face. *Stress* is commonly used to describe trivial irritations, but it's just as likely to be shorthand for more serious psychological challenges such as depression and anxiety. There is no single definition of *stress* that can encompass all these things, and yet we use that word to refer to all of them.

The fact that we use the word *stress* to describe so much of life is both a blessing and a curse. The downside is that it can make talking about the science of stress tricky. Even scientists—who usually nail down their definitions—use *stress* to describe a mind-boggling array of experiences and outcomes. One study might define it as feeling overwhelmed by caregiving demands, while another looks at it in terms of workplace burnout. One study uses *stress* to describe daily hassles, while another uses it to talk about the long-term effects of trauma. Worse yet, when this science gets communicated in the media, the headlines often use the familiar word *stress* but fail to provide details about what a study actually measured, leaving you to guess at whether the findings apply to your own life.

At the same time, there is a benefit to the catchall nature of the word. Because we use *stress* to describe so many aspects of life, how you think about it has a profound effect on how you experience life. Changing your thoughts about stress can have a similarly profound effect, transforming both everyday aggravations and how you relate to the biggest life challenges. So, rather than try to offer a narrow and manageable definition of *stress*, I'm willing to keep the meaning broad. Yes, it would be easier to say, "This book is about thriving under pressure at work" or "This book will help you manage the physical symptoms of anxiety." But the transformative power of choosing to see the upside of stress comes from its ability to change how you think about, and relate to, so many different aspects of life.

So as we begin this journey together, I offer this conception of stress: *Stress is what arises when something you care about is at stake.* This definition is big enough to hold both the frustration over traffic and the grief over a loss. It includes your thoughts, emotions, and physical reactions when you're feeling stressed, as well as how you choose to cope with situations you'd describe as stressful. This definition also highlights an important truth about stress: Stress and meaning are inextricably linked. You don't stress out about things you don't care about, and you can't create a meaningful life without experiencing some stress.

My goal, in writing this book, is to provide science, stories, and strategies that address the full range of what we mean by *stress*, even knowing that not every example will resonate with you, and that it is impossible to address every aspect of human experience that gets labeled as "stressful." We'll look at academic stress, work stress, family stress, health stress, financial stress, and social stress, as well as the challenges of dealing with anxiety, depression, loss, and trauma— things that might be best described as *suffering*, but that come up whenever I invite people to think about the stress in their own lives. I've also included the voices of my students to tell you how they have applied the ideas in this book. I've changed the names and some identifying details of those who wished to stay anonymous. But know that these are real stories from real people who hope that by shar- ing their experiences, they will help you have a different experience of stress. You'll also feel their presence throughout the book in the questions and concerns I try to address. I am grateful to them for helping me learn more about what it means to embrace stress in cir- cumstances far different from my own.

I trust you to pay the most attention to the science and stories that fit your life right now. The same applies to the exercises and strategies in the book. Just as no scientific study applies to all forms of stress, no one strategy for dealing with stress applies to every situation. A strat- egy that allows you to overcome public-speaking anxiety or better handle family conflict may not be the one that best helps you deal with financial problems or manage grief. I encourage you to choose the methods that seem best suited to your own challenges.

Whenever I talk about the upside of stress, someone always asks, "But what about the *really* bad stress? Does what you're saying still apply?" It's easy for people to see how embracing the small stress—some pressure at work, a little nervousness about a major event—could help. But what about the big stuff? Does the concept of embracing stress apply to trauma, loss, health problems, and chronic stress?

I can't guarantee that every idea in this book is going to help with every form of stress or suffering. However, I no longer worry that the benefits of embracing stress apply only to the small stuff. To my surprise, embracing stress has helped me the most in the most difficult situations—dealing with the death of a loved one, coping with chronic pain, and even overcoming a paralyzing fear of flying. That's also what I've heard from my students. The stories they share at the end of the course usually aren't about getting better at juggling deadlines or dealing with an irritating neighbor. They are about coming to terms with the loss of a spouse. Facing a lifelong struggle with anxiety. Making peace with a past that includes childhood abuse. Losing a job. Getting through cancer treatment.

Why would seeing the good in stress help in these circumstances? I believe it is because embracing stress changes how you think about yourself and what you can handle. It is not a purely intellectual exercise. Focusing on the upside of stress transforms how you experience it physically and emotionally. It changes how you cope with the challenges in your life. I wrote this book with that specific purpose in mind: to help you discover your own strength, courage, and compassion. Seeing the upside of stress is not about deciding whether stress is either all good or all bad. It's about how choosing to see the good in stress can help you meet the challenges in your life.

Rethink
STRESS

how to change your mind about stress

I STOOD IN THE Behavioral Research Lab at Columbia University holding my right arm out at shoulder height. Psychologist Alia Crum was trying to push it down. We struggled for a few seconds. Despite being quite petite, she was surprisingly strong. (I later learned that Crum had actually played Division I ice hockey in college and is currently an internationally ranked Ironman triathlete.)

My arm gave out.

"Now, instead of resisting me, I want you to imagine that you are reaching your arm toward someone or something you care about," Crum said. She asked me to imagine that when she pushed on my arm, I could channel her energy into what I was reaching toward. The exercise was inspired by her father, who is a sensei in aikido, a martial art based on the principle of transforming harmful energy. I visualized what Crum had instructed, and we tried again. This time, I was much stronger, and she wasn't able to push my arm down. The more she pushed, the stronger I felt.

"Were you really trying as hard this time?" I asked.

Crum beamed. She had just demonstrated the single idea that

motivates all her research: How you think about something can transform its effect on you.

I was meeting Crum in her basement lab at the Columbia Business School to talk about her research on stress. For a young scientist, Crum has an unusual track record of high-profile findings. Her work gets attention because it shows that our physical reality is more subjective than we believe. By changing how people think about an experience, she can change what's happening in their bodies. Her findings are so surprising that they make a lot of people scratch their heads and say, "Huh? Is that even possible?"

This reaction—*Is that even possible?*—is a familiar one to researchers who study *mindsets*. Mindsets are beliefs that shape your reality, including objective physical reactions (like the strength of my arm as Crum pushed on it), and even long-term health, happiness, and success. More important, the new field of mindset science shows that a single brief intervention, designed to change how you think about something, can improve your health, happiness, and success, even years into the future. The field is full of remarkable findings that will make you think twice about your own beliefs. From placebos to self-fulfilling prophecies, perception matters. After this crash course in the science of mindsets, you'll understand why your beliefs about stress matter—and how you can start to change your own mind about stress.

The Effect You Expect Is the Effect You Get

"Thinking Away the Pounds" and "Believe Yourself Healthy" were just two of the headlines that heralded the publication of one of Alia Crum's earliest studies. Crum had recruited housekeepers at seven hotels across the United States for a study of how beliefs affect health and weight. Housekeeping is strenuous work, burning over 300 calories an hour. As exercise, that puts it on par with weight lifting, water aerobics, and walking at 3.5 miles per hour. In comparison, office work—such as sitting in meetings or working on a computer—burns roughly 100 calories an hour. And yet, two-thirds of the housekeepers Crum recruited believed they weren't exercising regularly. One-third said they got no exercise at all. Their bodies reflected this perception. The average housekeeper's blood pressure, waist-to-hip ratio, and body weight were exactly what you'd expect to find if she were truly sedentary.

Crum designed a poster that described how housekeeping qualified as exercise. Lifting mattresses to make beds, picking towels off the floor, pushing heavily loaded carts, and vacuuming—these all require strength and stamina. The poster even included the calories burned while doing each activity (for example, a 140-pound woman would burn 60 calories cleaning bathrooms for fifteen minutes). At four of the seven hotels, Crum communicated this information to the housekeepers in a fifteen-minute presentation. She also hung copies of the poster, in both English and Spanish, on the bulletin boards in the housekeepers' lounges. Crum told them that they were clearly meeting or exceeding the surgeon general's recommendations for physical exercise and should expect to see the health benefits of being active. The housekeepers at the other three hotels were a control group. They received information about how important physical exercise is for health, but they were *not* told that their work qualified as exercise.

Four weeks later, Crum checked in with the housekeepers. Those who had been informed that their work was exercise had lost weight and body fat. Their blood pressure was lower. They even liked their jobs more. They had not made any changes in their behavior outside work. The only thing that had changed was their perception of themselves as exercisers. In contrast, housekeepers in the control group showed none of these improvements.

So, does this mean that if you tell yourself that watching television burns calories, you can lose weight? Sorry, no. What Crum told the housekeepers was true. The women really were exercising. Yet when she met them, they didn't see their work that way. Instead, they were more likely to view housekeeping as hard on their bodies.

Crum's provocative hypothesis is that when two outcomes are possible—in this case, the health benefits of exercise or the strain of physical labor—a person's expectations influence which outcome is more likely. She concluded that the housekeepers' perception of their work as healthy exercise transformed its effects on their bodies. In other words, *the effect you expect is the effect you get.*

Crum's next headline-making study pushed this idea further. The "Shake Tasting Study" invited hungry participants to come to the laboratory at eight in the morning after an overnight fast. On their first visit, participants were given a milkshake labeled "Indulgence: Decadence You Deserve," with a nutritional label showing 620 calories and 30 grams of fat. On their second visit, one week later, they drank a milkshake labeled "Sensi-Shake: Guilt-Free Satisfaction," with 140 calories and zero grams of fat.

As the participants drank the milkshakes, they were hooked up to an intravenous catheter that drew blood samples. Crum was measuring changes in blood levels of ghrelin, also known as the hunger hormone. When blood levels of ghrelin go down, you feel full; when blood levels go up, you start looking for a snack. When you eat something high in calories or fat, ghrelin levels drop dramatically. Less-filling foods have less impact.

One would expect a decadent milkshake and a healthful one to have a very different effect on ghrelin levels—and they did. Drinking the Sensi-Shake led to a small decline in ghrelin, while consuming the Indulgence shake produced a much bigger drop.

But here's the thing: The milkshake labels were a sham. Both times, participants had been given the same 380-calorie milkshake.

There should have been no difference in how the participants' digestive tracts responded. And yet, when they believed that the shake was an indulgent treat, their ghrelin levels dropped three times as much as when they thought it was a diet drink. Once again, the effect people expected—fullness—was the outcome they got. Crum's study showed that expectations could alter something as concrete as how much of a hormone the cells of your gastrointestinal tract secrete.

In both the housekeeping and the milkshake studies, when people's perceptions changed, their bodies' responses changed. And in each study, one particular belief seemed to enhance the body's most adaptive response: Viewing physical labor as exercise helped the body experience the benefits of being active. Viewing a milkshake as a high-calorie indulgence helped the body produce signals of fullness.

As interesting as weight loss and hunger hormones were, Crum was curious what other outcomes might be influenced by how we view things. Is there a perception that shapes our health in even bigger ways? She began to wonder about stress. She knew that most people view stress as harmful, even though it can also be beneficial. That's two possible effects. Could the effect that stress has on your well-being be determined, in part, by which effect you expect? And if Crum could change how a person thought about stress, would that change the way the person's body responded?

THAT QUESTION is why I found myself in Alia Crum's laboratory on a sunny morning in April. After I took the stairs down to the windowless basement and exchanged some pleasant introductions with the lab team, one of Crum's graduate students strapped me into what an outside observer might suspect was torture equipment. Two bands of metallic tape were wrapped tightly around my rib cage, and two around my neck. The bands were attached to an impedance cardiography machine that measured the activity of my heart. One blood pressure cuff squeezed my left bicep, while another gripped the index finger of my left hand. Electrodes on my inner elbow, fingertips, and leg measured blood flow and sweating. A thermometer attached to my right pinkie finger kept track of my body temperature. Then a lab assistant asked me to drool into a tiny test tube so that my saliva could be analyzed for stress hormones.

I was here to experience for myself what participants in Crum's most recent study had gone through. The goal of the study was to manipulate participants' views of stress and then watch how their bodies responded to a stressful situation.

The stress I was about to face was a mock job interview. To help me get better at interviewing, the mock interviewers would give me feedback as we went along. But this wasn't ordinary role-play. To make it extra stressful, the interviewers were trained to give me (and every other participant) negative feedback no matter what I said or did. My eye contact was poor. I picked a bad example. I uttered too many "uhs" and "ums." My posture suggested that I lacked confidence. They asked tough questions, like "Do you think gender inequality at the workplace is still a problem?" No matter what I or any participant said, the evaluators criticized the answers. Even though I knew that the whole thing was a carefully scripted experiment designed to throw me off balance, it was still stressful.

Before the mock job interview, every study participant was randomly assigned to view one of two videos about stress. The three-minute video I got opened with the message, "Most people think that stress is negative . . . but actually research shows that stress is enhancing." The video went on to describe how stress can improve performance, enhance well-being, and help you grow. The other video, which half the participants in the study watched, started with the ominous announcement, "Most people know that stress is negative . . . but research shows that stress is even more debilitating than you expect."

The video went on to describe how stress can harm your health, happiness, and performance at work.

Both videos cited real research, so in this sense they were both true. But each video was designed to activate a specific perception of stress—one that Crum hoped would influence how participants' bodies responded to the stress that followed.

I went through this mock experiment months after Crum had finished conducting the study. That meant that as soon as I finished the job interview and the electrodes came off, I got to hear the preliminary results. One finding blew me away.

The saliva I had drooled into the test tube provided a sample of two stress hormones: cortisol and dehydroepiandrosterone (DHEA). These hormones are both released by your adrenal glands during times of stress, but they serve different roles. Cortisol helps turn sugar and fat into energy and improves the ability of your body and brain to use that energy. Cortisol also suppresses some biological functions that are less important during stress, such as digestion, reproduction, and growth. DHEA, on the other hand, is a neurosteroid, which is exactly what it sounds like: a hormone that helps your brain grow. In the same way that testosterone helps your body grow stronger from physical exercise, DHEA helps your brain grow stronger from stressful experiences. It also counters some of the effects of cortisol. For example, DHEA speeds up wound repair and enhances immune function.

You need both of these hormones, and neither is a "good" nor "bad" stress hormone. However, the ratio of these two hormones can influence the long-term consequences of stress, especially when that stress is chronic. Higher levels of cortisol can be associated with worse outcomes, such as impaired immune function and depression. In contrast, higher levels of DHEA have been linked to a reduced risk of anxiety, depression, heart disease, neurodegeneration, and other diseases we typically think of as stress-related.

The ratio of DHEA to cortisol is called the *growth index* of a stress response. A higher growth index—meaning more DHEA—helps people thrive under stress. It predicts academic persistence and resilience in college students, as well as higher GPAs. During military survival training, a higher growth index is associated with greater focus, less dissociation, and superior problem-solving skills, as well as fewer post-traumatic stress symptoms afterward. The growth index even predicts resilience in extreme circumstances, such as recovering from child abuse.

Crum wanted to see if changing people's perceptions of stress could modify this measure of resilience. Could a three-minute video about stress alter this key ratio of stress hormones?

The answer, amazingly, is yes.

The videos had no effect on cortisol levels. Everyone's cortisol went up during the mock interview, as expected. However, participants who had watched the stress-is-enhancing video before the interview released more DHEA and had a higher growth index than participants who had watched the stress-is-debilitating video. Viewing stress as enhancing made it so—not in some subjective, self-reported way, but in the ratio of stress hormones produced by the participants' adrenal glands. Viewing stress as helpful created a different biological reality.

From Placebo to Mindset

One way to think about Crum's stress study is that it demonstrated a placebo effect. The positive stress video changed participants' expectations of how stress would affect them and, like a sugar pill, produced the expected response.

The placebo effect is a powerful phenomenon, but it's also a manipulation. Someone is telling you how to think about something. Often, they are giving you something you don't have any preconceived notions about. They hand you a pill and say, "This will help," so you believe them. But when it comes to stress, everyone already has a point of view. Every time you experience stress, your beliefs about it come to mind. Think about how many moments of your day you would describe as stressful. How often do you say, "This is so stressful" or "I'm so stressed"? In each of these moments, how you think about stress can alter your biochemistry and, ultimately, how you respond to whatever has triggered the stress.

A belief with this kind of power goes beyond a placebo effect. This is a mindset effect. Unlike a placebo, which tends to have a short-lived impact on a highly specific outcome, the consequences of a mindset snowball over time, increasing in influence and long-term impact.

As we've seen, a mindset is a belief that biases how you think, feel, and act. It's like a filter that you see everything through. Not every belief can become a mindset. Some beliefs simply aren't that important. You might believe that chocolate is better than vanilla, that it's rude to ask somebody's age, and that the world is round, not flat. Those beliefs, no matter how strongly you hold them, have relatively little consequence for how you think about your life.

The beliefs that become mindsets transcend preferences, learned facts, or intellectual opinions. They are core beliefs that reflect your philosophy of life. A mindset is usually based on a theory about how the world works. For example, that the world is getting less safe, that money will make you happy, that everything happens for a reason, or that people cannot change. All of these beliefs have the potential to shape how you interpret experiences and make decisions. When a mindset gets activated—by a memory, a situation you find yourself in, or a remark someone makes—it sets off a cascade of thoughts, emotions, and goals that shape how you respond to life. This, in turn, can influence long-term outcomes, including health, happiness, and even longevity.

Take, for example, how you think about growing older. As I mentioned before, having a positive view of aging adds an average of almost eight years to one's life. It predicts other important health outcomes, too. For example, the Baltimore Longitudinal Study of Aging, which tracked adults ages eighteen to forty-nine for an impressive thirty-eight years, found that those with the most positive views of aging had an 80 percent lower risk of heart attack. Beliefs about aging also influence recovery from major illnesses and accidents. In one study, adults who associated growing older with positive stereotypes such as "wise" and "capable" recovered from a heart attack more quickly than those who endorsed negative stereotypes such as "useless" and "stuck in their ways." In another study, a positive view of aging predicted faster and more complete physical recovery from a debilitating illness or accident. Importantly, both studies measured recovery in objective outcomes, such as walking speed, balance, and ability to perform daily activities. (By the way, if these findings make you want to adopt a more positive view of aging, consider this: Studies consistently show that people get happier as they get older, even though younger adults find this difficult to believe.)

How exactly does a belief about aging—sometimes measured decades earlier—affect heart attack rates, disability, and the risk of dying? The studies all controlled for important factors such as initial health status, depression, and socioeconomic status, so these do not explain the effects.

Instead, one likely answer is health behaviors. People with a negative view of aging are more likely to view poor health as inevitable. Because they feel less capable of maintaining or improving their health as they age, they invest less time and energy in their future well-being. In contrast, people with a positive attitude toward growing older engage in more health-promoting behaviors, like exercising regularly and following their doctor's advice. Changing a person's mind about aging can even promote healthy behaviors. For example, an intervention designed to increase positive views of aging also increased participants' physical activity. When you have a positive view of growing older, you're more apt to do things that will benefit your future self.

Beliefs about aging have an especially big impact on behaviors following a major health challenge. Researchers at the German Centre of Gerontology in Berlin followed older adults over time to examine the impact of a serious illness or accident, such as a broken hip, lung disease, or cancer. Those with a positive view of aging responded to the crisis by increasing their commitment to their health. They were more proactive and dedicated to their recovery. In contrast, older adults who had a more negative view of aging were less likely to take actions to improve their health. These choices, in turn, influenced recovery. Participants with a more positive view of aging ended up reporting greater life satisfaction, as well as better physical health and physical function, after their illness or accident.

How you think about aging can even influence your will to live as you grow older. People who hold negative views of aging when they are middle-aged report less of a will to live later in life. As older adults, they are more likely to view their lives as empty, hopeless, or worthless. In one study, Yale psychologists tested the effects of beliefs about aging on the will to live by subliminally priming older adults with either negative or positive stereotypes about aging. The researchers then asked the older adults to make hypothetical medical decisions. Older adults who had been primed with positive stereotypes were more likely to agree to a life-prolonging intervention for a potentially fatal illness. In contrast, those exposed to negative stereotypes were more likely to reject treatment.

Findings like this suggest that how you think about aging affects health and longevity not through some mystical power of positive thinking but by influencing your goals and choices. This is a perfect example of a mindset effect. It is more powerful than a placebo effect because it doesn't just alter your present experience but also influences your future.

It turns out that how you think about stress is also one of those core beliefs that can affect your health, happiness, and success. As we'll see, your stress mindset shapes everything from the emotions you feel during a stressful situation to the way you cope with stressful events. That, in turn, can determine whether you thrive under stress or end up burned out and depressed. The good news is, even if you are firmly convinced that stress is harmful, you can still cultivate a mindset that helps you thrive.

What Is Your Stress Mindset?

Psychologist Alia Crum and her colleagues developed the Stress Mindset Measure to assess people's views of stress. Take a moment to look at the two stress mindsets below and consider which set of statements you agree with more strongly—or, at least, would have agreed with before you picked up this book:

Mindset 1: Stress Is Harmful.
    Experiencing stress depletes my health and vitality.
    Experiencing stress debilitates my performance and productivity.
    Experiencing stress inhibits my learning and growth.
    The effects of stress are negative and should be avoided.

Mindset 2: Stress Is Enhancing.
    Experiencing stress enhances my performance and productivity.
    Experiencing stress improves my health and vitality.

Experiencing stress facilitates my learning and growth.

The effects of stress are positive and should be utilized.

Of these two mindsets, "stress is harmful" is by far the most common. Crum and her colleagues have found that while most people can see some truth in both mindsets, they still view stress as more harmful than helpful. Men and women do not differ, and age does not predict mindset.

The trends Crum has observed are consistent with the findings of other U.S. surveys. In a 2014 survey conducted by the Robert Wood Johnson Foundation and the Harvard School of Public Health, 85 percent of Americans agreed that stress has a negative impact on health, family life, and work. According to the American Psychological Association's Stress in America survey, most people perceive their own stress levels as unhealthy. Even those who report relatively little stress believe that the ideal level of stress is below whatever they are currently experiencing. Over the years, people's perceptions of a healthy level of stress have actually gone down; when the American Psychological Association started its annual stress survey in 2007, people perceived a moderate level of stress as ideal. Now, survey participants perceive that same moderate level of stress as unhealthy.

However, there is also evidence that people can see some good in stress. In 2013, I conducted a survey of CEOs, vice presidents, and general managers who were participating in Stanford University's Executive Leadership Development program, and 51 percent said they did their best work while under stress. In the 2014 Harvard School of Public Health survey, 67 percent of those who reported the highest levels of stress also said they had experienced at least one benefit from their stress. However, participants in both surveys were also convinced that they should be doing more to reduce stress. This attitude toward stress isn't an exclusively American mindset. I've encountered similar views about stress in Canada, Europe, and Asia. Even when people can recognize some benefits of stress, their overall perception of it is strongly negative.

Importantly, a negative view of stress is associated with very different outcomes than a positive perspective. Crum's research shows that people who believe stress is enhancing are less depressed and more satisfied with their lives than those who believe stress is harmful. They have more energy and fewer health problems. They're happier and more productive at work. They also have a different relationship to the stress in their lives: They are more likely to view stressful situations as a challenge, not an overwhelming problem. They have greater confidence in their ability to cope with those challenges, and they are better able to find meaning in difficult circumstances.

Now, if you're like me, your first response to these findings is skepticism. I think my first response went something like this: "People who have a positive view of stress are happier and healthier because they aren't actually stressed. The only way you end up with a positive view of stress is if you haven't had enough stress in your life yet. Suffer a little more, and then your opinion about stress will change."

Although my skepticism was motivated more by my own stress mindset than by scientific high-mindedness, it's still a reasonable hypothesis. Crum considered the possibility that a positive view of stress might be the result of an easier life. But when she looked at the data, she found only a weak link between how people thought about stress and the severity of the stress they were under. She also found a very small correlation between the number of stressful life events (such as divorce, the death of a loved one, or changing jobs) that people experienced in the past year and how negative their views of stress were. It is *not* the case that people with a positive attitude toward stress have a life free of suffering. Moreover, Crum also found that a positive view of stress was beneficial to people whether they were currently under a little or a lot of stress, and no matter how stressful or stress-free the past year had been.

Maybe, then, your stress mindset isn't so much a reflection of how much stress you've experienced but rather some kind of fixed personality trait. After all, some people are more likely to take a positive view of everything, stress included. And research shows that optimists live longer than pessimists. Maybe it's this general optimism that protects people from the harmful effects of stress. Crum considered this, too. It turns out that people with a stress-is-enhancing mindset are more likely to be optimists, but the correlation is small. In addition to optimism, two other personality traits seem to be associated with a more positive view of stress: mindfulness and the ability to tolerate uncertainty. However, Crum's analyses showed that none of these personality traits could account for the effects of stress mindset on health, happiness, or work productivity. While how a person thinks about stress might be influenced by certain personality traits or experiences, a stress mindset's effects on health and happiness cannot be explained by either.

Crum's research points to a more likely possibility: Stress mindsets are powerful because they affect not just how you think but also how you act. When you view stress as harmful, it is something to be avoided. Feeling stressed becomes a signal to try to escape or reduce the stress. And indeed, people who endorse a stress-is-harmful mindset are more likely to say that they cope with stress by trying to avoid it. For example, they are more likely to:

- Try to distract themselves from the cause of the stress instead of dealing with it.
- Focus on getting rid of their feelings of stress instead of taking steps to address its source.

- Turn to alcohol or other substances or addictions to escape the stress.
- Withdraw their energy and attention from whatever relationship, role, or goal is causing the stress.

In contrast, people who believe that stress can be helpful are more likely to say that they cope with stress proactively. For example, they are more likely to:

- Accept the fact that the stressful event has occurred and is real.
- Plan a strategy for dealing with the source of stress.
- Seek information, help, or advice.
- Take steps to overcome, remove, or change the source of stress.
- Try to make the best of the situation by viewing it in a more positive way or by using it as an opportunity to grow.

These different ways of dealing with stress lead to very different outcomes. When you face difficulties head-on, instead of trying to avoid or deny them, you build your resources for dealing with stressful experiences. You become more confident in your ability to handle life's challenges. You create a strong network of social support. Problems that can be managed get taken care of, instead of spiraling out of control. Situations that you can't control become opportunities to grow. In this way, as with many mindsets, the belief that stress is helpful becomes a self-fulfilling prophecy.

The First Stress Mindset Intervention

To truly test the effects of a stress mindset, you have to change someone's mind about stress and follow them over time. That's exactly what Crum and her colleagues did next.

The first stress mindset intervention took place at the global financial firm UBS during the height of the 2008 economic collapse. The financial industry is a notoriously stressful place to work. One study found that within ten years of entering the industry, 100 percent of investment bankers developed at least one condition associated with burnout, such as insomnia, alcoholism, or depression. The 2008 economic collapse only amplified the pressure. Financial workers reported significantly greater workplace stress, fear of layoffs, exhaustion, and burnout. Across the industry, there were widespread reports of increased anxiety, depression, and suicide.

Like most financial firms, UBS was hit hard. According to its 2008 annual report, shareholders experienced a 58 percent drop in the value of their shares. UBS instituted major layoffs and cut employee compensation by 36 percent. In the middle of all this, employees at UBS received an email from human resources inviting them to participate in a stress-management program. A total of 388—half men and half women, with an average age of thirty-eight—signed up. These stress-mindset guinea pigs were dealing with an increased workload, uncontrollable work demands, and enormous uncertainty about their own futures. So, yes, they knew stress.

The employees were randomly assigned to one of three groups. The first group, with 164 employees, received an online training that delivered the typical stress-management message, which reinforces the view that stress is inherently negative. The second group, with 163 employees, received an online training designed to give them a more positive view of stress; this was the mindset intervention. A smaller control group of 61 employees got no training at all.

Over the course of one week, employees in the online trainings received emails with links to three videos that were each three minutes long. Those in the first group were treated to statistics like "Stress is America's number one health issue" and "Stress is linked to the six leading causes of death." The videos warned that stress can lead to mood swings, emotional exhaustion, and memory loss. The videos also featured examples of leaders who failed to perform well under stress.

Employees in the mindset intervention group watched three very different videos. These videos explained how stress can increase physical resilience, enhance focus, deepen relationships, and strengthen personal values. The videos shared examples of companies that thrived under difficult circumstances, as well as people who performed heroically in the face of great stress.

All the employees completed surveys before and after the online trainings. The answer to the research team's first question—Can you change a person's mind about stress?—was yes. Employees who watched the negative videos became even more convinced that stress was harmful. In contrast, employees in the mindset intervention group developed a more positive view of stress.

How big was this mindset shift? Not huge. The employees did not suddenly forget everything they had ever heard about how harmful stress is. They were not begging for more stress. But they did endorse a view of stress that was more balanced than the one they'd had before the intervention. The change was statistically significant, but it wasn't a complete reversal. Instead of viewing stress as predominantly harmful, they now saw both the good and the bad in stress.

The second important question is whether this mindset shift was associated with any other changes. The answer again was yes. Employees who received the mindset intervention were less anxious and depressed. They reported fewer health problems, like back pain and insomnia. They also reported greater focus, engagement, collaboration, and productivity at work. Crucially, these improvements took place in the midst of extreme stress. Employees who watched the negative videos, as well as those who received no training, showed no change in these outcomes.

Crum has gone on to conduct stress mindset interventions and workshops in a variety of settings, including with health care professionals, college students, executives, and even Navy SEALs. She has also experimented with other methods for changing people's stress mindsets, some of which we'll see later in this chapter. What her work shows is that very brief interventions can lead to lasting changes in how people think about and experience stress. Adopting a more positive view of stress reduces what we usually think of as stress-related problems and helps people thrive under high levels of stress.

These findings, like the results of Crum's early research, might leave you scratching your head, wondering how exactly this works. To understand why mindset interventions can have such strong effects—and how you might begin to change your own mind about stress—let's take a closer look at what science tells us about the art of changing minds.

The Art of Changing Mindsets

Greg Walton, a psychologist at Stanford University, is, like Alia Crum, a mindset master. He's spent the past decade perfecting the art of changing minds with brief, one-dose interventions that have a major impact. His interventions—often lasting only one hour—produce improvements in everything from marital satisfaction to GPAs, physical health, and even willpower. In some cases, the results of that one hour persist years after the intervention. As part of his passion for translating scientific findings into meaningful change, Walton has presented his work at the White House, and, through Stanford's Center for Social Psychological Answers to Real-World Questions, has helped create a catalog of evidence-based solutions to guide policymakers, educators, and organizations in applying psychological science to real-world problems.

In each of his interventions, Walton targets one belief that research shows can get in the way of well-being or success—for example, the notion that intelligence is a fixed trait that cannot be developed. He creates a brief intervention that offers an alternative perspective and helps participants try on that new way of thinking. That's it. The whole approach is: Here's an idea you might not have considered. How do you think it applies to you? Then he follows people over time to see how the idea takes root.

When I asked Walton what his favorite mindset intervention was, he immediately pointed to one that he conducted on a group of freshmen at an Ivy League school. In this study, Walton delivered a simple message: If you feel like you don't belong, you aren't alone. Most people feel that way in a new environment. Over time, this will change.

Walton selected social belonging as his focus because he knew that the sense of *not* belonging—at school, at a workplace, or in any community that matters to you—is widespread. However, few people express it openly. Most people think they are the only ones who feel like they don't fit in.

Feeling like you don't belong can change how you interpret everything you experience. Conversations, setbacks, misunderstandings— almost anything can be viewed as evidence that, in fact, you don't belong. The belief that you don't belong also feeds into many destructive states of mind, from impostor syndrome (*I'm a fraud, and everyone will find out*) to stereotype threat (*Everyone expects to me to fail*) and self-handicapping (*Why bother trying?*). These states of mind can lead to self-destructive behaviors like avoiding challenges, hiding your problems, ignoring feedback, and not forming supportive relationships. Such behaviors, in turn, increase the risk of failure and isolation, which are taken as proof that you didn't belong after all. It's a self-fulfilling prophecy that Walton hoped to interrupt by changing how the Ivy League freshmen thought about their feelings of not belonging.

In the first part of the mindset intervention, Walton had the freshmen read excerpts from a survey of juniors and seniors discussing their experiences at the school. All the excerpts were chosen to communicate the message that everyone struggles with social belonging, but that this changes with time. For example, one senior wrote:

> When I first got here, I worried that I was different from other students. I wasn't sure I fit in. Sometime after my first year, I came to realize that many people come here uncertain whether they fit in or not. Now it seems ironic. Everybody feels they are different freshman year from everybody else, when really in at least some ways we are all the same.

After students read the survey excerpts, the experimenter asked them to write an essay reflecting on how their own experiences at college were similar to those described by the seniors and juniors. When the students were done writing, the experimenter explained that the school was creating an infomercial to show during next year's freshman orientation. The video was intended to help the arriving students understand what to expect in college. The experimenter asked the students if they would be willing to read their essays in front of a video camera, so they could be included in the infomercial. "As you probably know, it can be difficult to come into a new situation not knowing what to expect, and you, as an older student who has just gone through the same experience, are in a great position to help these freshmen out," the experimenter explained. "Do you think you would be able to do this?"

That's the entire intervention. Students read a survey, wrote an essay, and gave a message of social belonging to next year's freshmen.

The first time this intervention was offered, Walton tracked its effects on African American students, who have typically struggled the most with feelings of not belonging at the Ivy League school. The results were astonishing. The onetime intervention improved the students' academic performance, physical health, and happiness over the next three years, compared with students who had not been randomly selected to receive the intervention. By graduation, their GPAs were significantly higher than the GPAs of African American students who hadn't participated. In fact, their GPAs were so high that they had completely closed the typical GPA gap between minority and non-minority students at the school.

When Walton looked at what might explain these outcomes, he found that the intervention had changed two things. First, it changed the way students responded to academic and social problems. They were more likely to view their problems as short-lived and part of the college experience. Second, the intervention influenced the students' social worlds. Students who received the mindset intervention were more likely to find a mentor and to form more close friendships. "The process begins in a psychological way," Walton told me, "but then it becomes sociological."

Walton and his colleagues have delivered the belonging intervention in many settings. In one study, it boosted college retention rates more than giving students a $3,500 scholarship did. In another, it reduced college dropout rates by half. When female engineering students received the intervention, they started to perceive the engineering department as more welcoming. They went on to develop more friendships with male engineers, and even reported hearing fewer sexist jokes. "Their social world is changing," Walton explains.

Perhaps the most remarkable thing about this kind of mindset intervention is that people typically forget it. At the final follow-up in his Ivy League study, when students were graduating, Walton asked them if they remembered participating in the study freshman year. While 79 percent remembered participating in some study, only 8 percent remembered what it was about. Instead, the new mindset had become part of how they thought about themselves, and about the school. They forgot the intervention, but they internalized the message.

I think this is one of the most promising aspects of mindset science. Once an idea takes root, you don't have to work so hard at it. It's not a conscious strategy you need to employ or an inner debate you need to have every day. After an initial introduction to a new mindset, it can take hold and flourish.

Walton acknowledges that, to many, these results sound more like science fiction than science. But mindset interventions are not miracles or magic. They are best thought of as catalysts. Changing your mindset puts into motion processes that perpetuate positive change over time.

Why Mindset Interventions Can Be Hard to Grasp

Psychologists who conduct mindset interventions are used to skepticism. It strikes many people as ridiculous to claim that a brief, one-time intervention, whose only content is a new way to *think* about something, could change someone's life. Even when mindset interventions succeed beyond researchers' wildest expectations, it's hard for people to believe they actually work.

David Yeager, a mindset researcher at the University of Texas at Austin, shared a story with me that reveals how deep people's skepticism can run. The intervention in this story took place at the second-lowest-income high school in the San Francisco Bay Area. The school had some of the lowest test scores in the state. Almost three-quarters of its students were eligible for a free school lunch. Many of them had gang affiliations, and 40 percent said they did not feel safe at school.

Yeager wanted to teach freshmen at this school a growth mindset—the belief that people can change in significant ways. To do this, he had the students read a short article that introduced a few key ideas: Who you are now is not necessarily who you will be later in life; how people treat you or see you now is not necessarily a sign of who you really are or who you will be in the future; people's personalities can change meaningfully over time. The students also read first-person accounts from upperclassmen describing experiences that reflected this message of change. Finally, the students were asked to write a story about their own experiences of how people—themselves included—could change over time.

Yeager administered this thirty-minute intervention at the beginning of the school year in the high school gym, to 120 ninth-graders in gym shorts. As the students were reading the first article, a member of the athletic staff, who did not know the details of the intervention, came over to Yeager. "Why are you here?" he asked. "Why don't you go to the elementary school? 'Cause it's too late for these kids. This is a waste of your time." Yeager laughed when he told this story, but it's obvious that it upset him. "It's just this terrible irony. I'm literally here to teach these kids that they can change."

Despite the staff member's pessimism, the intervention had a profound and lasting impact. At the end of the school year, students who had received the intervention were more optimistic and less overwhelmed by the problems in their lives. They had fewer health problems and were less likely to become depressed than students who had been randomly assigned to a control group. A full 81 percent of the students who received the intervention passed their ninth-grade algebra class, compared with only 58 percent of students in the control group. The effect of the intervention on academic achievement was strongest for those whose mindset had changed the most. On average, these students began freshman year with a 1.6 GPA (equivalent to a C–) and ended with a 2.6 GPA (B–).

Those outcomes were so impressive that I felt sorry for the kids who got randomly assigned to the control group. Surely, these results would have wowed the school and changed the staff member's attitude toward the students' potential. And yet, according to Yeager, results like this often fail to impress. Yeager always shows his data to the staff at the schools where he conducts a study. He's passionate about education, and before becoming a researcher, taught middle school English in Tulsa, Oklahoma. So he gives them all the materials they need to continue to offer the mindset intervention, but many schools fail to take any next step. According to Yeager, the idea that a thirty-minute intervention could alter the trajectory of a person's life is just too much for people to wrap their heads around. "People just don't believe it's real," he said.

That's the thing about mindset interventions: They seem too good to be true. They contradict a deeply held cultural belief about the process of change itself. We believe that all meaningful problems are deeply rooted and difficult to change. Many problems *are* deeply rooted, and yet one of the themes you'll see again and again in this book is that small shifts in mindset can trigger a cascade of changes so profound that they test the limits of what seems possible. We are used to believing that we need to change everything about our lives first, and then we will be happy, or healthy, or whatever it is we think we want to experience. The science of mindsets says we have it backward. Changing our minds can be a catalyst for all the other changes we want to make in our lives. But first, we may need to convince ourselves that such change is possible.

How to Change Your Mindset

When the video of my TED Talk on embracing stress, given in Edinburgh, Scotland, in June 2013, was first made public, I began to get one question more than any other: *How* can I change my mind about stress?

In the stress mindset interventions we've looked at so far, people were manipulated into a mindset shift. Nobody said, "Seeing the good in stress is good for you." The message was much simpler: "Stress *is* good for you." Can a mindset shift still work if you try to change your own mind about stress, or do you have to be tricked into it?

One way to answer this question is to go back to the placebo effect. For a long time, doctors and scientists thought the placebo effect required deception. A sugar pill would help only if patients were convinced they were taking a real drug. But it turns out that deception is not the active ingredient in placebos. They work even when patients know they are taking a placebo.

In open-label placebo trials, patients are handed a packet clearly labeled "Placebo." The ingredients list is short: microcrystalline cellulose (sugar). The doctor tells the patient that yes, this is a placebo, and no, there is no active ingredient in it. But, the doctor explains, your mind and body are capable of many healing processes on their own, and placebos can trigger those processes. The doctor encourages the patient to take the sugar pills on a regular basis.

Surprisingly, pills clearly labeled "Placebo" have provided relief from migraine headaches, irritable bowel syndrome, and depression, often with benefits comparable to the best real treatments. Asking patients to be in on the trick—by explaining how the placebo effect works—does not reduce the placebo's effectiveness. It may even enhance the effect.

Research on mindset interventions shows that the same can be true when it comes to choosing a new mindset. When people are told how a mindset intervention works and are encouraged to remember the new mindset in everyday life, it does not decrease its effectiveness.

Alia Crum, whose first stress mindset interventions used biased videos to influence participants' beliefs about stress, thinks the ideal mindset intervention is less about manipulation and more about choice. The approach she and her colleagues now take is more transparent than the training she used at UBS during the 2008 economic collapse. The new intervention teaches participants about the power of mindset and invites them to adopt a more positive view of stress.

The first test of this "open-label" mindset intervention took place at a Fortune 500 firm. Employees were invited to participate in a stress-management training, and 229 mostly middle-aged employees signed up. About half were randomly assigned to a two-hour stress mindset intervention, while the others were put on a wait list.

The training started by letting employees know about research on both the harms and the benefits of stress. Then the employees learned about the power of mindset, including the results of Crum's previous studies. The employees were explicitly told that the aim of the training was to help them choose a more positive stress mindset.

To help them cultivate this new mindset, the employees were asked to reflect on their own experiences with stress, including times when stress had been helpful. They were also taught a three-step process for practicing the new mindset whenever they felt stressed. The first step is to acknowledge stress when you experience it. Simply allow yourself to notice the stress, including how it affects your body. The second step is to welcome the stress by recognizing that it's a response to something you care about. Can you connect to the positive motivation behind the stress? What is at stake here, and why does it matter to you? The third step is to make use of the energy that stress gives you, instead of wasting that energy trying to manage your stress. What can you do right now that reflects your goals and values? The employees were encouraged to remember this three-step process when they experienced stress and to try to practice it at least once a day.

Three weeks later, the researchers checked in with the participants. Those who had gone through the training showed a shift in stress mindset. Before the training, the employees had generally endorsed a stress-is-harmful mindset, but now they were more likely to recognize its upside. They were also better at dealing with stress. The employees reported less anxiety and depression and better physical health. At work, they felt more focused, creative, and engaged. The employees whose mindset changed the most—from most negative to more positive—showed the biggest improvements. At a final follow-up six weeks after the intervention, these benefits were maintained.

By comparison, the employees who had been put on the wait list showed no such changes—until they went through the two-hour training themselves. Then they reported the same mindset changes and improvements as the first group. Importantly, none of these benefits could be explained by a reduction in the amount of stress the employees reported. The intervention did not reduce stress; it transformed stress.

THE MOST effective mindset interventions have three parts: 1) learning the new point of view, 2) doing an exercise that encourages you to adopt and apply the new mindset, and 3) providing an opportunity to share the idea with others. As we've seen, the new mindset is usually introduced with a bit of science or storytelling. This book, like my New Science of Stress course, follows this same three-step process. In fact, the six-week Stanford class is one big mindset intervention. I tell students at our very first meeting that I am going to try to change their minds about stress. Each week, I give a lecture on the science included in this book and suggest specific strategies for cultivating a new stress mindset. In the class meeting that follows, I ask the students to report back on the ideas we discussed the previous week. Were they able to use any of the strategies? Did rethinking stress help them handle a difficult situation? I also ask them to pay special attention to any opportunities to share what they are learning with others. Their last assignment is to report back on what they found most helpful and how they shared that idea or practice with someone they care about.

Anonymous class surveys before and after the course show that, on average, students' stress mindsets become more positive by the end of the course. In the follow-up survey, students are also less likely to agree with statements such as "My problems make it difficult for me to live a life that I value," and "If I could magically remove all the painful experiences I've had in my life, I would do so." This mindset shift is accompanied by other benefits. Students report feeling more confident in their ability to handle the stress in their lives and feeling less overwhelmed by the problems they face. They are also more likely to say that they are energetically pursuing the goals that are important to them. One of my favorite comments was from a student who wrote at the end of the course evaluations, "I am not nearly as afraid of stress as I was before." And all these changes occurred despite the fact that many of my students are horrified when they realize, in the first class session, that the course they signed up for is about embracing stress, not reducing it.

Students also let me know in the anonymous post-course evaluations how they are applying the new mindset in their lives. I have been surprised, and encouraged, to see the diversity of situations students feel better able to handle. One student had a son on active duty, assigned to a special-ops wing of the U.S. Air Force. There are times the family has no idea where he is. The student found the course helpful in dealing with the stress of separation and the uncertainty of not knowing. Another student had recently left a bad marriage and was starting over on her own. The new stress mindset reinforced her belief that she had the ability to move on, and gave her a more positive way to think about her past experience. Another student had recently been demoted at work, and had fallen into a pattern of doing less than his best and isolating himself from his coworkers. He had been telling himself that disengaging at work was helpful because it allowed him to avoid the stress he felt about being demoted. The class helped him realize how self-defeating that was, and he was able to re-engage in a more productive way on the job. These are just a few examples of the kinds of challenges my students were dealing with. The new mindset didn't change the situations themselves, but it did change the students' relationships to them. In my experience, when people are willing to contemplate a new way of thinking about stress, the benefits can extend to just about any scenario you can imagine.

Of course, that willingness isn't always there. As I know all too well, it can be incredibly difficult, and even threatening, to rethink a belief important enough to earn the status of *mindset*. If you are used to viewing stress as the enemy, you may find it difficult and disorienting to choose to see the good in it. This book, like my course, is designed to help you through the process, if you are willing. The Rethink Stress exercises you'll find in the next two chapters give you a chance to try on a new stress mindset, and the Transform Stress exercises you'll find in Part 2 take the process a step further by showing you how to apply these ideas in your own life. Since the last step in changing your mindset is to share the ideas that are most helpful to you with others, throughout the book I offer suggestions of how you might do this, whether by sharing a particularly fascinating study, talking about your personal challenges, or helping others embrace their own stress.

GET TO KNOW YOUR STRESS MINDSET

The first step toward changing your mind about stress is to notice how your current mindset shows up in everyday life. We usually don't see the effect of a mindset because we are too identified with the beliefs behind it. The mindset doesn't feel like a choice that we make; it feels like an accurate assessment of how the world works. Even if you are fully aware of what you think about stress, you probably don't realize how that belief affects your thoughts, emotions, and actions. I call this "mindset blindness." The solution is to practice mindset mindfulness—by paying attention to how your current stress mindset operates in your life.

To get to know your stress mindset, start to notice how you think and talk about stress. Because a mindset is like a filter that colors every experience, you'll probably discover that you have a standard way of thinking and talking about stress. What do you say out loud or think to yourself? (My own stressed-out mantra, before I started to seriously rethink stress, was "This is too much!") Notice how thinking about stress in your habitual way makes you feel. Does it motivate you? Inspire you? Exhaust you? Paralyze you? How does it make you feel about yourself or your life?

Your stress mindset will also influence how you react to other people's stress. Notice how you feel and what you say or do when people around you are stressed. When other people complain about stress, does it make you anxious? Do you tell them to calm down or not to stress so much? Do you try to avoid people when they are most frazzled? Or do you use other people's stress as an invitation to vent about your own problems, as if you were competing to see whose life is more stressful? Whatever you observe yourself doing, try to notice its effects. How does it affect your own well-being or influence your relationships with others?

Then, start to look for stress mindsets in the world around you. What are the messages you get on a daily basis about how you're supposed to think about stress? Once you start looking for stress mindsets, you'll see them everywhere: in the media, in how other people talk about their lives, even in advertisements that use the promise of stress reduction to sell everything from shampoo to office furniture. As I was working on this chapter, someone sent me an article titled "10 Reasons Why Stress Is the Most Dangerous

Toxin in Your Life"—and it turned out to be an advertorial for a holistic remedy. I don't know if the article boosted sales, but the title alone was a brilliant way to create some extra stress about stress. Notice how it affects you to hear messages like this. Do they motivate self-care, or do they just make you worry about your health? When other people talk about their stress from a certain mindset, how does it make you feel about your own stress?

Practicing mindset mindfulness doesn't require anything other than curiosity. You're just starting to get to know how beliefs about stress—your own and those of the people around you—influence how you feel and how you cope. As we move forward, you'll learn how to counter less helpful beliefs and to put a more positive mindset into action.

Final Thoughts

About a year ago, I confessed to Alia Crum that I sometimes still caught myself complaining, "I'm so stressed!" or "This is so stressful!" I had already publicly renounced a stress-is-harmful mindset, but the old way of thinking still crept in when I felt especially overwhelmed. I didn't know if I should feel guilty about this, and I asked Crum if her mindset transformation was more complete.

She thought for a moment and said, "Yes, I do sometimes still say, 'I'm so stressed,' but then I hear myself, and I take a moment to think about why I'm stressed. Then I say, 'Ahhh, I'm *so stressed*.'"

Now, I can't convey in words the tone of voice she said this in, but suffice it to say that it didn't sound anything like the desperate bleats of *my* version of "I'm so stressed." Instead, when she said those three words, she sounded uplifted. I laughed and asked Crum if she was serious. She was. And then she explained how, in her view, the most helpful mindset toward stress is one that is flexible, not black or white: to be able to see both sides of stress but choose to see the upside; to feel your own distress and yet also decide to focus on how that stress connects to what you care about. Her hunch is that making a deliberate shift in mindset when you're feeling stressed is even more empowering than having an automatically positive view.

To this end, it's important to note that in all the stress mindset interventions, including my course at Stanford, people don't report a completely overhauled view of stress. The benefits of a mindset shift appear as soon as people begin to see the upside of stress. It's not clear whether there is some kind of critical threshold or whether a bigger mindset shift always comes with bigger benefits. The most important takeaway, to me, is that seeing the good in stress doesn't require abandoning the awareness that, in some cases, stress is harmful. The mindset shift that matters is the one that allows you to hold a more balanced view of stress—to fear it less, to trust yourself to handle it, and to use it as a resource for engaging with life.

beyond fight-or-flight

I N THE LATE 1990s, an unusual experiment took place in the trauma center of an Akron, Ohio, hospital. Patients who had just survived a major car or motorcycle accident were asked to pee into a cup. These urine samples were part of a study on post-traumatic stress disorder (PTSD). The researchers wanted to know: Can you predict who develops PTSD based on their level of stress hormones immediately after the trauma?

One month after their accidents, nine of the fifty-five patients were diagnosed with PTSD. They had flashbacks and nightmares. They tried to avoid reminders of the accident by not driving, staying off highways, or refusing to talk about what happened. Yet forty-six patients were not suffering in the same way. These more resilient patients had a different post-accident pee profile than the patients who developed PTSD. They had *higher* levels of the stress hormones cortisol and adrenaline.

Cortisol and adrenaline are part of what scientists call the *stress response*, a set of biological changes that helps you cope with stressful situations. Stress affects many systems of your body, from your cardiovascular system to your nervous system. Although the purpose of these changes is to help you, the stress response—like stress in general—is more feared than appreciated. Most people view the stress response as a toxic state to be minimized, but the reality is not so bleak. In many ways, the stress response is your best ally during difficult moments—a resource to rely on rather than an enemy to vanquish.

The study of accident survivors at the Akron trauma center was just the first of several showing that a *stronger* physical stress response predicts better long-term recovery from a traumatic event. In fact, one of the most promising new therapies to prevent or treat PTSD is administering doses of stress hormones. For example, a case report in the *American Journal of Psychiatry* describes how stress hormones reversed post-traumatic stress disorder in a fifty-year-old man who had survived a terrorist attack five years earlier. After taking ten milligrams of cortisol a day for three months, his PTSD symptoms decreased to the point that he no longer became extremely distressed when he thought about the attack. Physicians have also begun to administer stress hormones to patients about to undergo traumatic surgery. Among high-risk cardiac surgery patients, this approach has been shown to reduce the time in intensive care, minimize traumatic stress symptoms, and improve quality of life six months after surgery. Stress hormones have even become a supplement to traditional psychotherapy. Taking a dose of stress hormones right before a therapy session can improve the effectiveness of treatment for anxiety and phobias.

If these findings surprise you, you aren't alone. Most people believe that the body's stress response is uniformly harmful. Stress hormones are seen as toxins to be eliminated, not as potential therapies to be explored. From the conventional point of view, your body betrays you every time your hands get clammy, your heart races, or your stomach twists into knots. To protect your health and happiness, the thinking goes, your number one priority should be to shut down the stress response.

If this is how you think about the stress response, it's time for an update. While the stress response can be harmful in some circumstances, there is also much to appreciate. Rather than fearing it, you can learn to harness it to support resilience.

In this chapter, we'll look at how stress got its bad reputation, and why you shouldn't believe every scary headline you read. We'll also explore the latest understanding of the biology of stress, including how your stress response helps you engage, connect, and grow. Finally, we'll debunk the view that your stress response is an outdated survival instinct. Far from being a burden left over from your animalistic past, the stress response helps you be fully human today.

How Stress Got Its Bad Reputation

The year was 1936, and Hungarian endocrinologist Hans Selye was injecting lab rats with a hormone isolated from a cow's ovaries. He hoped to identify the hormone's effects by watching what happened to the poor rodents. Unfortunately for the rats, the results were not pretty. The caged critters developed bleeding ulcers. Their adrenal glands ballooned, while their thymuses, spleens, and lymph nodes— all parts of the immune system—shriveled up. These were some sad, sick rats.

But was the cow hormone really to blame? Selye ran control experiments, injecting some rats with a salt solution and some with a hormone isolated from a cow's placenta. Those rats developed the same symptoms. He tried extracts made from kidneys and spleens. Those rats got sick, too. Anything he injected the rats with made them sick, in exactly the same way.

Eventually, Selye had a flash of insight: The rats weren't getting sick because of what they were injected with, but because of what they were experiencing. There was something inherently toxic about getting stuck with needles. Selye found that he could create the same symptoms by subjecting rats to any uncomfortable experience: exposing them to extreme heat or cold, forcing them to exercise without rest, blasting them with noise, giving them toxic drugs, even partially severing their spinal cords. Within forty-eight hours, the rats lost muscle tone, developed digestive ulcers, and entered immune system failure.

Then they died.

This is how the science of stress was born. Selye chose the word *stress* to describe both what he was doing to the rats (nowadays, we'd say he was stressing them out) and how their bodies reacted (what we call the stress response). What does all this have to do with you? Well, before taking up the noble profession of torturing rats, Selye had been a physician. In that time, he observed many patients whose bodies were falling apart. They were diagnosed with one disease but had other symptoms—loss of appetite, fever, fatigue—that weren't specific to that condition. They seemed worn-out and run-down. At the time, Selye called it "sick syndrome."

Years later, when Selye ran his laboratory experiments, the sick and dying rats reminded him of his old patients. Perhaps, he reasoned, the cumulative wear and tear of life's challenges weakened the body. Here is where Selye made the grand leap from rat experiments to human stress. He hypothesized that many conditions plaguing humans, from allergies to heart attacks, were the result of the process he had observed in his rats. Selye's leap from rats to humans was theoretical, not experimental. He had studied lab animals all his life. But that didn't keep him from speculating about humans. And with this leap in logic, Selye made one more decision that forever changed how the world thought about stress. He chose to define *stress* in a way that went far beyond his laboratory methods with rats. *Stress*, he claimed, was *the response of the body to any demand made on it.* It wasn't just a response to noxious injections, traumatic injuries, or brutal laboratory conditions, but to anything that requires action or adaptation. By defining *stress* in this way, Selye set the stage for our modern terror about stress.

Selye dedicated the rest of his career to spreading the word about stress. He toured the world teaching other physicians and scientists about *le stress, el stress, lo stress,* and *der stress.* He became known as the Grandfather of Stress and was nominated for the Nobel Prize ten times. He even penned what was probably the first official guide to stress management. Along the way, his work was funded by some unusual allies. The tobacco industry paid him to write papers about the harmful effects of stress on human health. Under the industry's direction, he even testified to the U.S. Congress that smoking was a good way to prevent the harmful effects of stress.

But what Selye really gave the world was the belief that stress is toxic. If you tell a coworker, "This project is giving me an ulcer," or complain to your spouse, "This stress is killing me," it's Selye's rats you're paying tribute to.

Was Selye wrong? Not exactly. If you're the human equivalent of Selye's rats—deprived, tortured, or abused—then, yes, your body will pay a price. There is ample scientific evidence that severe or traumatic stress can harm your health. However, Selye defined stress so broadly that it includes not just trauma, violence, and abuse, but also *just about everything that happens to you.* To Selye, *stress* was synonymous with the body's response to life. If this is your definition of the word, and you think that the inevitable consequence of stress is to end up like Selye's rats, then of course you'll be worried.

Selye eventually recognized that not all stressful experiences will give you ulcers. He started talking about good stress (*eustress*) as an antidote to bad stress (*distress*). He even tried to improve stress's image, saying in a 1970s interview, "There is always stress, so the only point is to make sure that it is useful to yourself and useful to others." But it was too late. Selye's work had already instilled a general fear about stress in the general public and the medical community.

THE LEGACY of Hans Selye lives on in stress research, which relies heavily on laboratory animals rather than human subjects. To this day, much of what you hear about stress's harmful effects comes from studies of lab rats. But the stress those rats suffer is not everyday human stress. If you are a lab rat, a stressful day might look like this: Unpredictable, uncontrollable electric shocks. Getting thrown into a bucket of water and forced to swim until you start to drown. Being put in solitary confinement, or housed in overcrowded cages with inadequate food to fight over. This isn't stress; this is *The Hunger Games* for rodents.

I recently attended a talk by a prominent researcher whose animal work has been widely used to explain how stress can lead to mental illness in humans. He told us how he induced stress in his lab mice. First, he selects mice bred to be smaller than the typical mouse. Then he puts a small mouse in a cage with a much bigger mouse bred for aggression. He lets the alpha mouse attack the smaller mouse for twenty minutes, then rescues it. The smaller, injured mouse is separated from the alpha mouse but housed in a new cage where it can smell and see the alpha mouse that attacked it. The physical danger is lifted, but the psychological terror persists. This procedure doesn't happen just once, but *every day*. For weeks, the smaller mouse is taken out of its cage and put back in the cage with the aggressive mouse for a daily dose of bullying. When the scientist considers the mouse sufficiently stressed, he looks at how the experience affected its behavior. (Remarkably, many of the abused mice show total resilience to the experience, although some develop what looks like the mouse equivalent of depression.)

I don't doubt that this research is an excellent model for some forms of human stress, including child abuse, domestic violence, and imprisonment—all of which can have devastating effects. But when headlines declare, "Science Proves Stress Makes You Depressed," the stories rarely consider whether the methods used to stress out lab animals are equivalent to what most people mean when they complain, "I'm so stressed." For some perspective, consider that in a major 2014 survey in the United States, the most commonly named source of daily stress among people who claimed to be highly stressed was "juggling schedules of family members." The runner-up was "hearing about what politicians are doing."

More often, the word *stress* is used to gloss over the study details, with no distinction between the effects of abuse and trauma and the effects of daily hassles. This results in a lot of unnecessary stress about stress. For example, when a friend of mine was pregnant with her first child, she saw a study online that put her in a panic. The headline warned that a mother's stress during pregnancy is passed on to the baby. My friend was under a lot of pressure at work, and she began to worry. Was she permanently harming her baby by not going on early maternity leave?

I encouraged her to take a deep breath. The study she had seen was done on rats, not humans. (Yes, I looked it up—what are friends for?) The rats' stress during pregnancy consisted of two things: daily restraint stress—a euphemism for putting an animal in a container no bigger than its body, with minimal holes for ventilation—and forced swimming, or making a rat tread water until it starts to drown. As much pressure as my friend felt at work, it was nothing like this.

When you look at human studies, it becomes clear that stress during pregnancy is not always harmful. A 2011 review of over a hundred studies found that only severe stress, such as surviving a terrorist attack or being homeless during pregnancy, increased the risk of preterm birth and low birth weight. Higher levels of daily stress and hassles did not. Some degree of stress during pregnancy may even benefit the baby. For example, researchers at Johns Hopkins University found that women who reported greater stress during pregnancy had babies born with superior brain development and higher heart rate variability, a biological measure of resilience to stress. The exposure to a mom's stress hormones in the womb teaches a baby's developing nervous system how to handle stress. So my friend needn't have panicked. Yes, she might have been passing her stress on to her baby—but that stress might have been making her baby resilient.

The message that all stress during pregnancy is harmful may even lead to unintended consequences. For example, one survey of women who drank alcohol during pregnancy found that it was viewed as an acceptable, even desirable way to reduce stress. As one woman told the researchers, "It's better for me if I drink, at least the stress is going away." When stress and anxiety are viewed as toxic states, we may turn to even more destructive behaviors in the attempt to protect ourselves or shelter those we care about.

Instead, we can take comfort in the research that shows how stressful experiences can themselves be protective. Stanford biopsychologist Karen Parker studies the effects of early life stress on both humans and squirrel monkeys. To stress out young monkeys, she separates them from their mothers and places them in an isolated cage for one hour a day. The separation is clearly distressing to the monkeys, but less inhumane than methods used in other animal research. In many ways, that makes it an excellent model for ordinary childhood stress.

When Parker first started separating the young monkeys from their moms, she predicted that the early life stress would lead to emotional instability. But instead, the stress led to resilience. As they grew up, the monkeys who had experienced early life stress were less anxious than the more sheltered monkeys. They explored more in new environments and showed greater curiosity toward new objects—a young monkey's version of courage. They were quicker to solve new mental challenges that the experimenters gave them. As juveniles—the equivalent of teenagers—the previously stressed monkeys even showed greater self-control. All of these effects lasted into adulthood. The early life stress had set the young monkeys on a different developmental trajectory, one characterized by greater curiosity and resilience.

Parker's research team has even looked at how early life stress changes the developing brain. The monkeys who had been separated from their moms developed larger prefrontal cortexes. In particular, early life stress beefed up regions of the prefrontal cortex that dampen fear responses, improve impulse control, and increase positive motivation. Parker and other scientists believe that childhood stress can also create similarly resilient brains in humans. Most important, this appears to be a natural part of the how the brain adapts to stress—not a rare occurrence or an uncommon outcome.

The science of stress is complex, and there is no doubt that some stressful experiences lead to negative outcomes. But we are not Selye's lab rats. The stress those animals were exposed to is the worst possible kind: unpredictable, uncontrollable, and completely devoid of meaning. As we'll see, the stress in our own lives rarely fits this description. Even in circumstances of great suffering, human beings have a natural capacity to find hope, exert choice, and make meaning. This is why in our own lives, the most common effects of stress include strength, growth, and resilience.

Is It Wrong to Have a Stress Response?

Hans Selye's rats are one reason stress has such a bad reputation, but you can also blame Walter Cannon's cats and dogs. Cannon, a physiologist at Harvard Medical School, first described the fight-or-flight response in 1915. He was interested in how fear and anger affected animals' physiology. His favorite methods for making his animals angry and scared included "covering the cat's mouth and nose with the fingers until a distress of breathing is produced" and putting cats and dogs in a room together to fight.

Cannon observed that, when threatened, animals release adrenaline and enter a state of heightened sympathetic activation. Their hearts race, their breathing quickens, and their muscles tighten—they become ready for action. Their digestion and other non-emergency physical functions slow or stop. The body prepares for battle by increasing energy reserves and mobilizing the immune system. All these changes kick in automatically during the struggle to survive.

The fight-or-flight survival instinct is not uniquely canine or feline; it is present in any species with a pulse. Fight-or-flight has saved many a life, animal and human. It has been conserved by nature for this reason, and we should be happy to have this instinct built into our DNA.

However, as many scientists have pointed out, fistfights and quick escapes are not ideal coping strategies for the situations humans deal with every day. How will a fight-or-flight response help you manage the misery of your commute or the threat of unemployment? What will happen if you flee your relationship, kids, or job every time things get hard? You can't punch a past-due mortgage payment, and you can't make yourself disappear every time there's a conflict at home or at work.

From this point of view, the stress response is an instinct you should suppress in all but the most physical of crises, like escaping a burning building or rescuing a drowning child. For all the other challenges you face, the stress response is a waste of energy that gets in the way of successful coping. This is the *mismatch theory* of the stress response—it worked out for our ancestors, but not for us. You, poor human, are crippled with a stress response that has little adaptive function in the modern world.

The mismatch theory of the stress response hinges on the idea that there is only one kind of stress response. As Stanford neuroscientist Robert Sapolsky explains in the documentary *Stress: Portrait of a Killer* (how's that title for a mindset message?), "You turn the stress response on because a lion has mauled you; you turn the stress response on because you're thinking about taxes." If you think that the body's response to stress is always fight-or-flight, then the stress response begins to look like evolutionary baggage. This is what many scientists argue.

So what's wrong with this point of view? Let's be clear: A stress response that supported only two survival strategies—throw a punch or run like hell—would truly be a mismatch for modern life. But the full picture of the human stress response turns out to be much more complex. Fleeing and fighting are not the only strategies your body supports. As with humans themselves, the stress response has evolved, adapting over time to better fit the world we live in now. It can activate multiple biological systems, each supporting a different coping strategy. Your stress response won't just help you get out of a burning building; it will also help you engage with challenges, connect with social support, and learn from experience.

BEYOND FIGHT-OR-FLIGHT

Let's pretend, for a moment, that you are on a game show called *The Trust Game*. The host gives you one hundred dollars. The other player—a total stranger to you—is given zero dollars. If you choose not to trust the stranger, that hundred dollars will be split between the two of you, leaving you both with fifty. If you choose to trust the other player, the next decision is up to him. If he chooses to be trustworthy, the prize is increased, and you each get two hundred dollars. If he chooses to be untrustworthy, the prize is still increased, but he gets everything, and you get nothing.

Would you choose to trust the stranger? And what if the roles were reversed—would you be generous or selfish if the stranger decided to trust you?

A real British game show, *Golden Balls*, works on this premise, testing the limits of people's trustworthiness and selfishness. Although the show has been criticized for encouraging sociopathic behavior, behavioral economist Richard Thaler found that 53 percent of players choose to trust and be trustworthy. (He considered this percentage surprisingly high, but economists are not known for their faith in people's altruism.)

The Trust Game is a popular tool of behavioral economists studying how different factors, including stress, influence decision-making. In one study, men were put through a stressful group task that forced them to compete with other participants in a mock job interview and tests of cognitive ability. It was designed to maximize two aspects of stress: the pressure to perform and the threat of being compared with others. Immediately afterward, the men were given the chance to play the Trust Game with a different set of strangers—none of whom had been part of the stressful group experience. How trusting and trustworthy do you think these men were, compared with men who had not been stressed-out?

You might expect the stressed-out men to be more aggressive or selfish, but the opposite was true. Men who had just gone through a stressful experience were 50 percent more likely to extend trust to a stranger and risk their full share of the winnings. They were also 50 percent more likely to be trustworthy, splitting the winnings with the stranger instead of keeping the money for themselves. The rate of trust and trustworthiness in a control group of men who hadn't been stressed was quite similar to that of contestants on *Golden Balls*—around 50 percent. In contrast, the men who were stressed-out showed unusually high rates of trust and trustworthiness—around 75 percent. Stress made the men prosocial.

Throughout the study, researchers tracked the men's physical stress responses. Men who had the strongest cardiovascular reactivity to stress were also the most likely to trust and be trustworthy in the game that followed. In other words, the stronger their hearts' response to stress, the more altruistic they became.

This finding shocks a lot of people. I've had students raise their hands to argue that the study's findings are impossible. If you believe that stress always produces a fight-or-flight response, these men's behavior makes no sense. They should be operating from a dog-eat-dog, competitive mentality, ready to take the money of any suckers who make the mistake of trusting them.

The reason this finding *is* possible is because there are many potential stress responses. Unlike what most people believe, there is no one uniform physical stress response that is triggered by all stressful situations. The specific cardiovascular changes, ratio of hormones released, and other aspects of a stress response can vary widely. Differences in your physical stress response can create very different psychological and social responses, an increase in altruism among them.

There are several prototypical stress responses, each with a different biological profile that motivates various strategies for dealing with stress. For example, a *challenge response* increases self-confidence, motivates action, and helps you learn from experience; while a *tend-and-befriend response* increases courage, motivates caregiving, and strengthens your social relationships. Alongside the familiar fight-or-flight response, these make up your stress response repertoire. To understand how stress can trigger these very different states, let's take a closer look at the biology of stress.

Stress Gives You Energy to Help You Rise to the Challenge

As Walter Cannon observed, a fight-or-flight stress response starts when your sympathetic nervous system kicks in. To make you more alert and ready to act, the sympathetic nervous system directs your whole body to mobilize energy. Your liver dumps fat and sugar into your bloodstream for fuel. Your breathing deepens so that more oxygen is delivered to your heart. And your heart rate speeds up to deliver the oxygen, fat, and sugar to your muscles and brain. Stress hormones like adrenaline and cortisol help your muscles and brain take in and use that energy more efficiently. In all these ways, your stress response gets you ready to face whatever challenges lie in front of you.

This part of the stress response can give you extraordinary physical abilities. There are countless news reports of so-called hysterical strength attributed to stress, including the story of two teenage girls in Lebanon, Oregon, who raised a three-thousand-pound tractor off their father, who was trapped underneath. "I don't know how I lifted it, it was just so heavy," one of the girls told reporters. "But we just did it." Many people have this kind of experience during stress: They don't know how they find the strength or courage to act. But when it matters most, their bodies give them the energy and will to do what's necessary.

The energy you get from stress doesn't just help your body act; it also fires up your brain. Adrenaline wakes up your senses. Your pupils dilate to let in more light, and your hearing sharpens. The brain processes what you perceive more quickly. Mind-wandering stops, and less important priorities drop away. Stress can create a state of concentrated attention, one that gives you access to more information about your physical environment.

You also get a motivation boost from a chemical cocktail of endorphins, adrenaline, testosterone, and dopamine. This side of the stress response is one reason some people enjoy stress—it provides a bit of a rush. Together, these chemicals increase your sense of confidence and power. They make you more willing to pursue your goals and to approach whatever is triggering the flood of feel-good chemicals. Some scientists call this the "excite and delight" side of stress. It's been observed both in skydivers falling out of planes and people falling in love. If you get a thrill out of watching a close game or rushing to meet a deadline, you know this side of stress.

When your survival is on the line, these biological changes come on strong, and you may find yourself having a classic fight-or-flight response. But when the stressful situation is less threatening, the brain and body shift into a different state: the *challenge response*. Like a fight-or-flight response, a challenge response gives you energy and helps you perform under pressure. Your heart rate still rises, your adrenaline spikes, your muscles and brain get more fuel, and the feel-good chemicals surge. But it differs from a fight-or-flight response in a few important ways: You feel focused but not fearful. You also release a different ratio of stress hormones, including higher levels of DHEA, which helps you recover and learn from stress. This raises the growth index of your stress response, the beneficial ratio of stress hormones that can determine, in part, whether a stressful experience is strengthening or harmful.

People who report being in a flow state—a highly enjoyable state of being completely absorbed in what you are doing—display clear signs of a challenge response. Artists, athletes, surgeons, video gamers, and musicians all show this kind of stress response when they're engaged in their craft or skill. Contrary to what many people expect, top performers in these fields aren't physiologically calm under pressure; rather, they have strong challenge responses. The stress response gives them access to their mental and physical resources, and the result is increased confidence, enhanced concentration, and peak performance.

Stress Makes You Social to Encourage Connection

Your stress response doesn't just give you energy. In many circumstances, it also motivates you to connect with others. This side of stress is primarily driven by the hormone oxytocin. Oxytocin has gotten a lot of hype as the "love molecule" and the "cuddle hormone" because it's released from your pituitary gland when you hug someone. But oxytocin is a much more complex neurohormone that fine-tunes your brain's social instincts. Its primary function is to build and strengthen social bonds, which is why it's released during those hugs, as well as sex and breastfeeding. Elevated levels of oxytocin make you want to connect with others. It creates a craving for social contact, be it through touch, a text message, or a shared beer. Oxytocin also makes your brain better able to notice and understand what other people are thinking and feeling. It enhances your empathy and your intuition. When your oxytocin levels are high, you're more likely to trust and help the people you care about. By making the brain's reward centers more responsive to social connection, oxytocin even amplifies the warm glow you get from caring for others.

But oxytocin is about more than social connection. It's also a chemical of courage. Oxytocin dampens the fear response in your brain, suppressing the instinct to freeze or flee. This hormone doesn't just make you want a hug; it also makes you brave.

Sounds like a good hormone, right? Some people have even suggested that we snort it to become better versions of ourselves, and you can actually buy oxytocin inhalers online. But oxytocin is as much a part of your stress response as the adrenaline that makes your heart pound. During stress, your pituitary gland releases oxytocin to motivate social connection. That means stress can help you be this "better" version of yourself, no snorting required.

When oxytocin is released as part of the stress response, it's encouraging you to connect with your support network. It also strengthens your most important relationships by making you more responsive to others. Scientists refer to this as the *tend-and-befriend response*. Unlike the fight-or-flight response, which is primarily about self-survival, the tend-and-befriend response motivates you to protect the people and communities you care about. And, importantly, it gives you the courage to do so.

When all you want is to talk to a friend or a loved one, that's the stress response encouraging you to seek support. When something bad happens and you think about your kids, your pets, your family, or your friends, that's the stress response encouraging you to protect your tribe. When somebody does something unfair and you want to defend your team, your company, or your community, that's all part of this prosocial stress response.

Oxytocin has one more surprise benefit: This so-called love hormone is actually good for cardiovascular health. Your heart has special receptors for oxytocin, which helps heart cells regenerate and repair from any micro-damage. When your stress response includes oxytocin, stress can literally strengthen your heart. This is quite different from the message we usually hear—that stress will give you a heart attack! There *is* such a thing as a stress-induced heart attack, typically triggered by a massive adrenaline surge, but not every stress response damages your heart. In fact, one of the most provocative studies I've seen found that stressing out rats before trying to chemically induce a heart attack actually *protected* them from heart damage. But when researchers gave the rats a drug that blocked oxytocin release, stress no longer protected their hearts. This study hints at one of the most surprising sides of stress: Your stress response has a built-in mechanism for resilience—one that motivates you to care for others while also strengthening your physical heart.

Stress Helps You Learn and Grow

The last stage of any stress response is recovery, when your body and brain return to a non-stressed state. The body relies on a pharmacy of stress hormones to help you recover. For example, cortisol and oxytocin reduce inflammation and restore balance to the autonomic nervous system. DHEA and nerve growth factor increase neuroplasticity so that your brain can learn from stressful experiences. Though you may have thought of stress hormones as something you need to recover from, in this case, it's the reverse. These hormones are built into the stress response because they help you recover physically and mentally. People who release higher levels of these hormones during a stressful experience tend to bounce back faster, with less lingering distress.

The stress recovery process isn't instantaneous. For several hours after you have a strong stress response, the brain is rewiring itself to remember and learn from the experience. During this time, stress hormones increase activity in brain regions that support learning and memory. As your brain tries to process your experience, you may find yourself unable to stop thinking about what happened. You might feel an impulse to talk with someone about it, or to pray about it. If things went well, you might replay the experience in your mind, remembering everything you did and how it worked out. If things went poorly, you might try to understand what happened, imagine what you could have done differently, and play out other possible outcomes.

Emotions often run high during the recovery process. You may find yourself too energized or agitated to calm down. It's not uncommon to feel fear, shock, anger, guilt, or sadness as you recover from a stressful experience. You may also feel relief, joy, or gratitude. These emotions often coexist during the recovery period and are part of how the brain makes sense of the experience. They encourage you to reflect on what happened and to extract lessons to help you deal with future stress. They also make the experience more memorable. The neurochemistry of these emotions render the brain more plastic—a term used to describe how capable the brain is of remodeling itself based on experience. In this way, the emotions that follow stress help you learn from experience and create meaning.

This is all part of how past stress teaches the brain and body how to handle future stress. Stress leaves an imprint on your brain that prepares you to deal with similar stress the next time you encounter it. Not every minor irritation will trigger this process, but when you go through a seriously challenging experience, your body and brain learn from it. Psychologists call this *stress inoculation*. It's like a stress vaccine for your brain. That's why putting people through practice stress is a key training technique for NASA astronauts, emergency responders, elite athletes, and others who have to thrive in highly stressful environments. Stress inoculation has been used to prepare children for emergency evacuations, train employees to deal with hostile work environments, and even help coach those with autism for stressful social interactions. It can also explain the findings of scientists like Stanford's Karen Parker, who has shown how early life stress can lead to later resilience.

Once you appreciate that going through stress makes you better at it, you may find it easier to face each new challenge. In fact, research shows that expecting to learn from a stressful experience can shift your physical stress response to support stress inoculation. As we saw in Alia Crum's study, viewing a video on stress's enhancing qualities increased participants' DHEA levels during and after a mock job interview. Other studies show that viewing a stressful situation as an opportunity to improve your skills, knowledge, or strengths makes it more likely that you will have a challenge response instead of a fight-or-flight response. This, in turn, increases the chance that you will learn from the experience.

The Stress Response Helps You Rise to the Challenge, Connect with Others, and Learn and Grow

How the Stress Response Helps You:	How You Know It's Happening
Rise to the Challenge	
• Focuses your attention	*You notice your heart pounding, your body sweating, or your breath quickening. You are mentally focused on the source of stress. You feel excited, energized, anxious, restless, or ready for action.*
• Heightens your senses	
• Increases motivation	
• Mobilizes energy	
Connect with Others	
• Activates prosocial instincts	*You want to be near friends or family. You notice yourself paying more attention to others, or are more sensitive to others' emotions. You feel a desire to protect, support, or defend the people, organizations, or values you care about.*
• Encourages social connection	
• Enhances social cognition	
• Dampens fear and increases courage	
Learn and Grow	
• Restores nervous system balance	*Even though your body is calming down, you still feel mentally charged. You replay or analyze the experience in your mind, or want to talk to others about it. A mix of emotions are usually present, along with a desire to make sense of what happened.*
• Processes and integrates the experience	
• Helps the brain learn and grow	

Rethink Stress: Rethink Your Stress Response

Bring to mind a recent experience that you would describe as stressful. Maybe it's an argument you had, a problem you faced at work, or a health scare. Then read the summary chart "The Stress Response Helps You Rise to the Challenge, Connect with Others, and Learn and Grow." Take a moment to consider which aspects of the stress response were present during or after your stressful experience. Did your body try to give you more energy? How do you know this—what sensations did you feel in your body? Did you seek out social contact or support? What did the impulse to connect feel like? Were you motivated to act or to protect or defend someone or something you care about? How did that motivation express itself? Did you replay the incident in your mind after it was over or talk to someone about it? What emotions were present afterward—or perhaps now, as you think about the experience? Take a few moments to describe, in writing, what you felt.

Before, you might have viewed the sweaty palms, need for moral support, or rumination afterward as excessive stress "symptoms." Maybe you saw them as signs that you weren't handling stress well. Can you choose to rethink these same symptoms as signs that your body and brain are helping you cope? If there is one part of your stress response that you particularly dislike or mistrust, consider what role it might play in helping you protect yourself, rise to a challenge, connect with others, or learn and grow. Take a few more moments to write about your experience from this point of view.

Choose Your Own Stress Response

The latest science shows that there is more than one way to experience stress. But what determines which kind of stress response you have in any given moment?

Different types of stressful situations typically provoke different responses. For example, social stress usually increases oxytocin more than other kinds of stress. That's good, because it motivates social connection. In contrast, performance stress is more likely to increase adrenaline and other hormones that give you energy and focus. That's also good, because it's what you need to do your best. Ideally, your responses will be flexible and fine-tuned, and your body will respond to each stressful situation in a way that best uses your resources. A trial lawyer about to give summary statements should have a challenge response. When she gets home, if her kids are fighting over her attention, a tend-and-befriend response will soothe them and herself. And if the fire alarm goes off in the middle of the night, a fight-or-flight response will get her and the rest of the family out of the house safely.

Your life history can also influence how you respond to stress. In particular, your early experiences with stress can have a strong effect on how your stress system functions as an adult. For example, adults who experienced a life-threatening illness in their youth tend to show a strong oxytocin response to stress. They learned early on to rely on others in times of stress, priming them to have a tend-and-befriend response. In contrast, adults who experienced abuse during childhood show a smaller oxytocin response to stress. They are more likely to have learned not to trust others in stressful times. As adults, they are primed to cope through the self-defense of a fight-or-flight response or the self-reliance of a challenge response.

Even your genes shape how you respond to stress. Some genes predispose people to enjoy the adrenaline rush of a stress response and seek out stressful stimulation. These same genes increase the tendency to have a competitive, fight-or-flight response. Other genes affect how sensitive you are to oxytocin, and therefore influence the tendency to have a tend-and-befriend response to stress. Your genetic profile even influences how strongly stress affects you. Some people are born more resilient to stress, which makes them less reactive to stressful circumstances and less easily changed—for better or worse—by stressful experiences. Other people are naturally more sensitive to stress. Paradoxically, this increases the likelihood of both negative outcomes from stress, such as depression or anxiety, and positive outcomes, such as heightened compassion and personal growth.

However, as we'll see, none of these genetic differences are destiny. They set up predispositions that interact with your life experiences and conscious choices. The stress response system is adaptive, constantly trying to figure out how to best handle whatever challenges you face. For example, becoming a parent can change your stress tendencies. Men who were once die-hard fight-or-flighters experience a drop in testosterone that suddenly unleashes their tend-and-befriend side when they become fathers. In contrast, life-threatening traumatic events can push the stress system in the opposite direction. Trauma creates a temporary expectation that the world is an unsafe place, and the brain and body prepare by priming a fight-or-flight response. It's important to recognize that these changes are strategic, not signs of a broken stress system. Although these adaptations have costs, they also have very practical benefits. More important, these adaptations are not permanent. Your brain and body continue to reshape themselves to help you face the most important challenges in your life. Even changes induced by traumatic events can be reversed through new life experiences and relationships.

Finally, you have a say in how your body responds to stress. Stress is a biological state designed to help you learn from experience. That means your stress response is extremely receptive to the effects of deliberate practice. Whatever actions you take during stress, you teach your body and brain to do spontaneously. If you want to respond to stress differently—to face challenges confidently, to stand up for yourself, to seek social support instead of withdrawing, to find meaning in your suffering—there is no better way to change your habits than to practice this new response during stress. Every moment of stress is an opportunity to transform your stress instincts.

STRESS AT 36,000 FEET

A student sent me the following story shortly after the last lecture in my New Science of Stress course. Reva and her husband, Lakshman, had taken the course together. After the last class, they flew to Australia to be with one of their daughters, who was expecting a baby.

Lakshman suffers from heart disease, and one of the symptoms is obstructive sleep apnea. He needs to use a continuous airway pressure machine on flights to maintain adequate oxygen. The machine has to be plugged in, and it takes up a lot of space—something that makes flying a very stressful experience for both of them. On this flight, the power outlet was on the ceiling, and the connection kept coming loose. Because it was a night flight, the plane was dark, which made it hard to see. Reva, who has knee replacements, had to climb on her seat to reconnect the machine. Trying to maneuver in the cramped row was painful. She felt her whole body responding to the stress.

This is exactly the kind of situation where most people would say a stress response is a problem. Reva and her husband had little control over the situation, and getting angry at the outlet, the flight attendants, or each other wasn't going to help. Fleeing was impossible— unless they had brought parachutes and planned to dismantle the emergency exit window. Not to mention that Lakshman was at high risk for a heart attack. He surely didn't need an adrenaline rush at 36,000 feet.

But Reva remembered that the stress response is more than fight-or-flight. She and her husband talked about the stress they were feeling. Instead of stressing about the stress, they imagined their bodies releasing oxytocin to help them support each other and to protect Lakshman's heart. Knowing about the social side of the stress response, Reva befriended the woman in the seat next to her. Connecting with their rowmate made the rest of the long journey much easier, as Reva no longer worried about disturbing her with her movements.

Reva and Lakshman also made a conscious choice to shift their mental focus from trying to fix an uncontrollable situation to thinking about why the flight itself was important. They talked about how this ordeal was part of something meaningful—going to see their daughter and soon-to-be-born grandchild. This helped them appreciate the journey, even with its discomfort.

I love this story because it is a simple example of how remembering the many aspects of a stress response can transform your experience of stress. In this case, focusing on social connection and meaning was the perfect strategy for enduring a long and uncomfortable flight. In other situations, where you have more control, it might be more helpful to remember that your stress response is giving you energy and encouraging you to act.

When you feel your body responding to stress, ask yourself which part of the stress response you need most. Do you need to fight, escape, engage, connect, find meaning, or grow? Even if it feels like your stress response is pushing you in one direction, focusing on how you *want* to respond can shift your biology to support you. If there is a side of the stress response you would like to develop, consider what it would look like in any stressful situation you are dealing with now. What would someone who is good at that side of stress think, feel, or do? Is there any way to *choose* that response to stress right now?

Final Thoughts

One of the main arguments of the mismatch theory of the stress response—which says that the body's response to stress is an outdated survival instinct—is that you should not have a stress response to anything that isn't a life-threatening emergency. Getting stressed is seen as a psychological flaw, a weakness to be corrected. This stems from the mistaken belief that every stress response is a full-throttle fight-or-flight response. A more complete picture of the biology of stress helps us understand why we have these responses throughout the day, and why these are not signs of a flaw at all. Rushing to get your kids ready for school, dealing with a difficult coworker, thinking about criticism you received, worrying about a friend's health— we have stress responses to all these things because we get stressed when something important to us is at stake. And most important, *we have stress responses to help us do something about it.*

We get stressed when our goals are on the line, so we take action. We get stressed when our values are threatened, so we defend them. We get stressed when we need courage. We get stressed so we can connect with others. We get stressed so that we will learn from our mistakes.

The stress response is more than a basic survival instinct. It is built into how humans operate, how we relate to one another, and how we navigate our place in the world. When you understand this, the stress response is no longer something to be feared. It is something to be appreciated, harnessed, and even trusted.

a meaningful life
is a stressful life

FROM 2005 TO 2006, researchers from the Gallup World Poll asked more than 125,000 people, ages fifteen and up, from 121 countries one question: Did you feel a great deal of stress yesterday? In industrialized nations, the pollsters conducted phone surveys, and in developing countries and remote regions, they went door-to-door.

Then the researchers computed an index of national stress. What percentage of a country's population said, yes, they felt stressed-out yesterday? Worldwide, the average was 33 percent. The United States came in high, at 43 percent. The Philippines took the top spot at 67 percent, and Mauritania ranked last at just over 5 percent.

Because country-by-country percentages varied, the researchers wondered: Does a nation's stress index correspond with other indexes of well-being, like happiness, life expectancy, and national GDP? Consider what your own beliefs about stress would predict. Is having more stressed-out people good for public health, national happiness, and the economy?

To the researchers' surprise, the higher a nation's stress index, the higher the nation's well-being. The higher the percentage of people who said they had felt a great deal of stress the day before, the higher that nation's life expectancy and GDP. A higher stress index also predicted higher national scores on measures of happiness and satisfaction with life. More people reporting stress meant more people satisfied with their health, work, standard of living, and community. The researchers also observed that people living in countries with high levels of corruption, poverty, hunger, or violence, such as Mauritania, didn't always describe their days as stressful. Whatever people around the world meant when they said they felt stressed, it did *not* correspond perfectly to what the researchers considered objectively bad societal conditions.

To understand this puzzling finding, the researchers looked at the relationship between stress and other emotions. On a day when a person felt a great deal of stress, that person was also more likely to have felt angry, depressed, sad, or worried. But living in a country with a high stress index was also associated with reporting feeling more joy, love, and laughter the previous day. When it came to overall well-being, the happiest people in the poll weren't the ones without stress. Instead, they were the people who were highly stressed but not depressed. These individuals were the most likely to view their lives as close to ideal. In contrast, the researchers reported that among individuals who appeared to be the most unhappy, experiencing high levels of shame and anger and low levels of joy, "there was a notable lack of stress."

I call this the *stress paradox*. High levels of stress are associated with both distress and well-being. Importantly, happy lives are not stress-free, nor does a stress-free life guarantee happiness. Even though most people view stress as harmful, higher levels of stress seem to go along with things we want: love, health, and satisfaction with our lives.

How can something that we experience as distressing be associated with so many good outcomes? The best way to understand the stress paradox is to look at the relationship between stress and meaning. It turns out that a meaningful life is also a stressful life.

Is Your Life Meaningful?

In 2013, researchers at Stanford and Florida State University asked a broad national sample of U.S adults, ages eighteen through seventy-eight, to rate how much they agreed with the statement "Taking all things together, I feel my life is meaningful." That may seem like a tall order, asking people to reflect on the entirety of their lives to determine whether or not it has meaning. And yet, most people, with a quick gut check, know whether or not this feels true. Perhaps you made your own inner assessment, just from reading the statement.

The researchers then looked at what distinguished people who strongly agreed with the statement from those who did not. What are the best predictors of a meaningful life?

Surprisingly, stress ranked high. In fact, every measure of stress that the researchers asked about predicted a greater sense of meaning in life. People who had experienced the highest number of stressful life events in the past were most likely to consider their lives meaningful. People who said they were under a lot of stress right now also rated their lives as more meaningful. Even time spent worrying about the future was associated with meaning, as was time spent reflecting on past struggles and challenges. As the researchers conclude, "People with very meaningful lives worry more and have more stress than people with less meaningful lives."

Why are stress and meaning so strongly linked? One reason is that stress seems to be an inevitable consequence of engaging in roles and pursuing goals that feed our sense of purpose. When people report the biggest sources of stress in their lives, topping the list are work, parenting, personal relationships, caregiving, and health. In two recent surveys, 34 percent of adults in the U.K. named having a baby as the most stressful experience of their lives, while 62 percent of highly stressed adults in Canada named work as their biggest source of stress.

Whenever you ask people about these stressful but meaningful roles, the stress paradox shows up. For example, the Gallup World Poll found that raising a child under eighteen significantly increases the chance that you will experience a great deal of stress every day— *and* that you will smile and laugh a lot each day. Entrepreneurs who say that they experienced a great deal of stress yesterday are also more likely to say that they learned something interesting that day. Rather than being a sign that something is wrong with your life, feeling stressed can be a barometer for how engaged you are in activities and relationships that are personally meaningful.

Research also shows that a less stressful life doesn't make people nearly as happy as they think it will. Although most people predict they would be happier if they were less busy, the opposite turns out to be true. People are happier when they are busier, even when forced to take on more than they would choose. A dramatic *decrease* in busyness may explain why retirement can increase the risk of developing depression by 40 percent. A lack of meaningful stress may even be bad for your health. In one large epidemiological study, middle-aged men who reported higher levels of boredom were more than twice as likely to die of a heart attack over the next twenty years. In contrast, many studies show that people who have a sense of purpose live longer. For example, in a study that followed over nine thousand adults in the U.K. for ten years, those who reported highly meaningful lives had a 30 percent reduction in mortality. This reduced risk held even after controlling for factors including education, wealth, depression, and health behaviors such as smoking, exercise, and drinking.

Findings like this can help explain why stress is not always harmful for health and happiness—and why we should not fear leading stressful lives. When the most commonly reported sources of stress in people's lives overlap with the greatest sources of meaning, it's clear that stress may even contribute to well-being.

Stress may be a natural byproduct of pursuing difficult but important goals, but that doesn't mean every stressful moment is rich in meaning. And yet even when the stress we're under doesn't seem inherently meaningful, it can trigger the desire to *find* meaning—if not in this moment, then in the broader context of our lives. Far from being a luxury, the ability to find meaning in our lives helps us stay motivated in the face of great difficulties. Human beings have an innate instinct and capacity to make sense out of their suffering. This instinct is even part of the biological stress response, often experienced as rumination, spiritual inquiry, and soul-searching. Stressful circumstances awaken this process in us. This is one more reason why a stressful life is often a meaningful life; stress challenges us to find the meaning in our lives.

Rethink Stress: What Brings Meaning to Your Life?

Take a few moments to list your most meaningful roles, relationships, activities, or goals. In what parts of your life are you most likely to experience joy, love, laughter, learning, or a sense of purpose? When you have listed a few, ask yourself this: Would you also describe any of them as sometimes or frequently stressful?

We often imagine how ideal it would be to get rid of the stress we experience at home, at work, and in pursuit of our goals. But that isn't a realistic possibility. We don't get to choose between a stress-*full* or a stress-*free* experience of family, work, community, love, learning, or health. If there is something in your life that is both meaningful and causing you a great deal of stress, take a few moments to write about *why* this role, relationship, activity, or goal is so important to you. You might also consider writing about what life would be like if you suddenly lost this source of meaning. How would you feel about the loss? Would you want it back in your life?

FINDING THE MEANING IN EVERYDAY STRESS

Between 1961 and 1970, about thirteen hundred men living in the Boston area enrolled in the Veterans Affairs Normative Aging Study. Over the next five decades, the men reported on two types of stress in their lives: major life events (like getting a divorce or being in a serious accident) and the number of daily hassles they faced. In 2014, a major report was released that looked at the effects of stress on mortality among these men. Of the two types of stress, daily hassles were by far the better predictor of mortality. Men who reported the most daily hassles between 1989 and 2005 were three times more likely to have died by 2010 than those who reported the fewest hassles.

Naturally, the media headlines announced "Stressed Out Men Die Sooner" and "Stress Can Kill You, Science Says." But to understand what was toxic about their stress, you need to look at how the researchers measured what they called daily hassles. What was killing the men wasn't so much the presence of everyday stress, but their attitude toward it.

The Daily Hassles and Uplifts Scale lists fifty-three aspects of a typical life, including "your spouse," "the nature of your work," "the weather," "cooking," and "church or community organizations." It asks you to rate how much of a *hassle* each item was that day, as well as how much of an *uplift* it was. Basically, the scale asks whether you view the roles, relationships, and activities of your life as irritating inconveniences or meaningful experiences. You might think, "It depends on the day." But actually, people's scores on this scale are remarkably stable over time. Feeling burdened rather than uplifted by everyday duties is more a mindset than a measure of what is going on in your life.

Importantly, how you think about stress can influence this tendency. When you believe that stress is harmful, anything that feels a bit stressful can start to feel like an intrusion in your life. Whether it's waiting in line at the grocery store, rushing to meet a deadline at work, or planning a holiday dinner for your family, everyday experiences can start to seem like a threat to your health and happiness. You may find yourself complaining about these experiences, as if your life has gone off course and there is some stress-free version of it out there waiting for you. Consider that in a 2014 survey by the Harvard School of Public Health, the most commonly named sources of everyday stress included juggling schedules, running errands, commuting, social media, and household tasks such as cooking, cleaning, and repairs. These are normal and expected parts of life, but we treat them as if they are unreasonable impositions, keeping our lives from how they should really be.

It was *this* mindset—not some objective measure of stressful events—that best predicted the risk of death among the men in the Normative Aging Study over five decades. Summing up the study as "stress kills" (which plenty of media reports did) doesn't make sense. The study's takeaway shouldn't be to try to reduce the so-called hassles in your life. The takeaway should be to change your relationship to the everyday experiences you perceive as hassles. The same experiences that give rise to daily stress can also be sources of uplift or meaning—but we must choose to view them that way.

A CLASSIC study from the 1990s points to one of the best ways to cultivate a mindset of meaning in everyday stress. A bunch of

Stanford students agreed to keep journals over winter break. Some were asked to write about their most important values, and how the day's activities related to those values. Others were asked to write about the good things that happened to them. After the three-week break was over, the researchers collected the students' journals and asked them about their breaks. The students who had written about their values were in better health and better spirits. Over break, they had experienced fewer illnesses and health problems. Heading back to school, they were more confident about their abilities to handle stress. The positive effect of writing about values was greatest for those students who had experienced the most stress over break.

The researchers then analyzed more than two thousand pages from the students' journals to see whether they could tell what had made the writing assignment so helpful. Their conclusion: Writing about values helped the students see the meaning in their lives. Stressful experiences were no longer simply hassles to endure; they became an expression of the students' values. Giving a younger sibling a ride reflected how much a student cared about his family. Working on an application for an internship was a way to take a step toward future goals. To the students asked to see their deepest values in daily activities, small things that might otherwise have seemed irritating became moments of meaning.

Since that first study, dozens of similar experiments have followed. It turns out that writing about your values is one of the most effective psychological interventions ever studied. In the short term, writing about personal values makes people feel more powerful, in control, proud, and strong. It also makes them feel more loving, connected, and empathetic toward others. It increases pain tolerance, enhances self-control, and reduces unhelpful rumination after a stressful experience.

In the long term, writing about values has been shown to boost GPAs, reduce doctor visits, improve mental health, and help with everything from weight loss to quitting smoking and reducing problem drinking. It helps people persevere in the face of discrimination and reduces self-handicapping. In many cases, these benefits are a result of a onetime mindset intervention. People who write about their values once, for ten minutes, show benefits months or even years later.

Why is this one small mindset intervention so powerful? Stanford psychologists Geoffrey Cohen and David Sherman analyzed over fifteen years' worth of studies on this mindset intervention and concluded that the power of writing about values is in how it transforms how you think about stressful experiences and your ability to cope with them. When people are connected to their values, they are more likely to believe that they can improve their situation through effort and the support of others. That makes them more likely to take positive action and less likely to use avoidant coping strategies like procrastination or denial. They also are more likely to view the adversity they are going through as temporary, and less likely to think that the problem reveals something unalterably screwed up about themselves or their lives.

Over time, this new mindset builds on itself, and people begin to see themselves as the kind of person who overcomes difficulties. Cohen and Sherman call this a "narrative of personal adequacy." In other words, when you reflect on your values, the story you tell yourself about stress shifts. You see yourself as strong and able to grow from adversity. You become more likely to approach challenges than to avoid them. And you are better able to see the meaning in difficult circumstances.

As with many effective mindset interventions, people often completely forget the experiment that sparked the positive changes. But the benefits persist because the story people tell themselves about stress has changed. The lasting benefits are not the direct result of the ten-minute writing period that happened long ago, but of the mindset shift that it inspired.

Rethink Stress: What Are Your Values?

The list of values below is not exhaustive, but it's designed to get you thinking about your own. Which values on the list are most important to you? Pick your top three, and if something comes to mind that is not on this list, write it down.

Acceptance	Fairness	Love
Accountability	Faith/Religion	Loyalty
Adventure	Family	Mindfulness
Art or Music	Freedom	Nature
Athletics	Friendship	Openness
Celebration	Fun	Patience
Challenge	Generosity	Peace/Nonviolence
Collaboration	Gratitude	Personal Growth
Commitment	Happiness	Pets/Animals
Community	Hard Work	Politics
Compassion	Harmony	Positive Influence
Competence	Health	Practicality
Cooperation	Helping Others	Problem-Solving
Courage	Honesty	Reliability
Creativity	Honor	Resourcefulness
Curiosity	Humor	Self-Compassion
Discipline	Independence	Self-Reliance
Discovery	Innovation	Simplicity/Thrift
Efficiency	Integrity	Strength
Enthusiasm	Interdependence	Tradition
Equality	Joy	Trust
Ethical Action	Leadership	Willingness
Excellence	Lifelong Learning	Wisdom

Once you've chosen three values as personally meaningful, pick one and write about it for ten minutes. Describe why this value is important to you. You could also write about how you express this value in your everyday life, including what you did today. If you are facing a difficult decision, you could write about how this value might guide you.

These ten minutes can change how you relate to the stress in your life, even if you don't write about anything that is currently stressful. You may want to repeat this exercise with the other two important values at another sitting, or revisit this exercise when you are feeling especially overwhelmed by stress.

Students sometimes tell me they struggle with choosing a value for this exercise—either they aren't sure how to identify their own values or they have difficulty narrowing it down to one. Keep in mind that values reflect what you care about. For this exercise, you are simply expressing what feels important and meaningful to you right now. It can be an attitude, a personal strength, a priority, or even a community you care about. It can be what you would like to experience in life or what you would like to share with others. It could be a principle you would like to use to make important life decisions.

For this exercise, it doesn't matter if you are "good" at a value, or if other people will understand why it is important to you. A value can be something that comes naturally to you or something that you would like to develop in yourself. For example, one of my students initially found this exercise uninspiring because she had picked competence— something that other people valued in her but that she didn't connect with emotionally. In fact, it was something she felt that other people expected of her, but that she herself resented. When I mentioned that she could choose something she aspired to, she realized that she wanted to cultivate greater acceptance, even though it was incredibly difficult for her.

REMEMBER YOUR VALUES

Sometimes when you are in the middle of a stressful situation, you need to shift your mindset. Research shows that reflecting on your values in moments of stress can help you cope. In a study at the University of Waterloo in Ontario, for example, participants were given bracelets that said, "Remember the values." In another version of this study, conducted at Stanford University, participants were given a keychain, instead of a bracelet, and wrote their personal values on a slip of paper that could be inserted into the keychain. The study participants were encouraged to look at the bracelet or keychain when they were feeling stressed and to think about their most important values in that moment. This added instruction helped people deal with adversity even better than a onetime writing exercise.

In my New Science of Stress course, I give all my students bracelets to remind them of their values. One of my students, Miriam, wrote to me about how it was helping her deal with an increasingly difficult situation. Her husband, Joe, appeared to be in the early stages of Alzheimer's disease. Though the diagnosis was tentative, Joe's neurologist had shared his suspicions that Alzheimer's was behind Joe's memory lapses. Joe was a former executive, and the first signs of his cognitive decline alarmed both Joe and Miriam. They had looked forward to growing old together, but the future they had imagined for themselves now seemed to be slipping away.

Miriam and Joe did the values exercise together. She chose patience as her most important value. Joe chose having a sense of humor and honesty. Miriam told me that she was able to remember and practice patience many times over the week. She also witnessed, and took strength from, Joe relying on his values. When Joe lost his cellphone and Miriam found it in the refrigerator, Joe admitted that he had no memory of leaving it there, and even joked about it. This lightened the moment of stress for both of them.

For Miriam and Joe, avoiding the stress wasn't possible, and denying it wasn't helpful. There wasn't much they could do to control the situation. Choosing their values was a way to take charge of at least one aspect of the experience. When you can't control or get rid of stress, you can still choose how you respond it. Remembering your values can help transform stress from something that is happening against your will and outside your control to something that invites you to honor and deepen your priorities.

Consider creating a physical reminder of your own most important value. Maybe it's not a bracelet or keychain, but a Post-it attached to your computer monitor or a sticker you put on your phone. Then, when stress hits, remember your value and ask yourself how it can guide you in this moment.

How We Talk About Stress

Two physicians sit across from each other. One says, "Tell me about a time when you were present for a patient in a moment of deep sadness." Then he listens in silence as the other physician, a clinical geneticist, recounts her story. She describes the experience of telling a woman in her forties that her sixteen-year-old son has Marfan syndrome, a rare genetic disorder that leads to abnormal bone development. People with the disorder tend to have very long limbs, fingers, and toes. It also weakens the heart. The woman's husband had died two years earlier from an aortic rupture due to Marfan syndrome. And the physician had to explain to this woman that her son carried the genetic defect that had killed his father.

When she is finished describing the experience, the listener gently probes, "What made that a memorable or meaningful experience?" And then, "What personal strengths did you bring to that moment that helped you respond to the suffering that was present?"

These physicians are participating in a program developed at the University of Rochester School of Medicine and Dentistry designed to reduce burnout in medical professionals. The program was developed by two physicians: Mick Krasner, who practices primary care internal medicine, and Ronald Epstein, a professor of family medicine, psychiatry, and oncology. They recognized the need for medical professionals to process the stress of their work. Many physicians have been trained to shut down the part of themselves that responds emotionally to pain, suffering, and death. To protect themselves from feeling too much, they may come to see patients as objects or procedures, rather than as human beings.

While this may initially seem like a good way to reduce stress, it comes with a heavy cost. For health care providers, deriving meaning from their work requires reflecting on the profound privilege of being with a person who is suffering and doing their best to relieve it. Trying to defend against the suffering around them can, paradoxically, increase their risk of burnout, by removing an important source of meaning. This problem is not unique to medical professionals. It is shared by those in law enforcement, social work, and education, as well as parents, caregivers, and clergy members. These roles can be exhausting, but they are also rich sources of personal meaning. Trying to create a psychological shield to defend against stress can interfere with the ability to find purpose and satisfaction.

Krasner and Epstein came up with a somewhat radical strategy for increasing physician resilience: Teach them to be more fully present, even in difficult moments. Embrace the relationship between suffering and meaning, rather than defend against it. Most important, create a community of fellow physicians who share and support a meaning-making mindset.

Once a week, a small group of physicians meet for two hours. They begin by practicing a mindfulness technique, such as awareness of breathing and body sensations. Unlike what many people think, mindfulness isn't about relaxation or escaping the stress of the day. Instead, it is the ability to pay attention to and accept whatever thoughts, sensations, and emotions are happening. If you're feeling sad, you notice what sadness feels like in your body. You don't try to push it away and replace it with happy thoughts. One of the effects of the biological stress response is to make you more open to your experience. You feel things more, and your ability to notice expands. You are more sensitive to other people and to your environment. This increased openness is helpful, but can be overwhelming. Many people, when they experience this opening in the presence of other people's suffering, want to slam it shut. So they distract themselves, or distance themselves, or get drunk. Mindfulness exercises are a way to practice staying open to what you sense and feel, rather than shutting down.

After the mindfulness practice, the physicians tell stories. At each meeting, a theme is offered. One week, they talk about a profound moment of caring for someone who is dying. The next, they share stories about a surprising clinical encounter that changed how they thought about a patient. Another week, the theme is mistakes, blame, and forgiveness. Storytelling extends an invitation to reflect on the challenges of practicing medicine—and the meaning that comes from them.

The physicians start by spending a few minutes on their own, writing some thoughts about a story they are willing to share. Then they get into pairs or small groups. One at a time, they tell their stories. The listeners have two jobs. First, to really listen—to let themselves hear, feel, and understand what the other person experienced—while noticing how this person's story affects them: how they feel when they listen, what judgments they make, what emotions surface. Their second job is to help the storyteller find meaning in the experience. The listeners do this by asking questions rather than giving advice. *What made that memorable? What did you do that helped in this situation? What did you learn about yourself?*

They are encouraged to bring the listening skills they develop in the group into their medical practice as well. Instead of rushing or shutting down, they can allow themselves to really hear, and feel, what a patient or family member is saying. To make eye contact and give patients and their families their full attention. To not interrupt, except to ask questions that help them understand the patient's experience. As they learned to do with one another in the storytelling exercises, the physicians practice opening up, rather than putting up a shield, during the stressful moments of their work.

The first seventy primary care physicians who completed this program met once a week for two months, then once a month for ten months. At the end of the program, they reported significantly less burnout. They were less emotionally drained from their work and less likely to dread getting up in the morning to face another day on the job. They found more satisfaction in their work, and were less likely to say that they regretted going into medicine. The physicians also felt less isolated in their stress. As one reflected, "That feeling that we're not alone, it validates what we're feeling, and what we're experiencing."

The improvement in the physicians' mental health was dramatic. Before the intervention, the physicians completed a survey of depression and anxiety. In a typical adult population, the average score for men is 15, and the average score for women is 20. The physicians' average score at the start of the study was 33. By the end of the first eight weeks, their score had dropped to 15. By the end of the one-year program, the average score was 11—a remarkable shift in psychological well-being, despite no change in the stressful nature of their work.

The physicians also felt increased empathy for patients. They described feeling curious about, instead of resentful toward, patients with difficult cases. They were more likely to feel grateful rather than overwhelmed when spending time with patients who were suffering.

Opening up to the suffering that is an intrinsic part of their work helped these physicians reconnect meaning to it. This is a strategy that challenges how we usually think about managing stress. Rather than trying to reduce stress, they embraced it. When stress is part of what makes something meaningful, shutting it out doesn't get rid of the stress. Instead, taking the time to fully process and make meaning from what is stressful can transform it from something that drains you into something that sustains you.

THIS APPROACH has helped me deal with stress in the professional role that I find most meaningful: teaching. One example stands out—an experience that haunted me but ultimately came to play an important role in my understanding of myself as a teacher. In 2006, I took over coordinating Stanford's Introduction to Psychology course, which enrolls hundreds of students, uses over a dozen teaching assistants, and includes guest lectures from many faculty members. It's a huge course to manage. After fall quarter, I felt like things had gone well for my first time. But then, in January 2007, I received an email from the academic director of an undergraduate residence hall. He informed me that one of my students from fall quarter, who had taken an incomplete in the course, had died over winter break.

I wasn't told how he had died, but I had a sinking feeling. I Googled his name and found two items. The first was a local news report from the previous summer, honoring him as his high school's valedictorian and describing his goal to study medicine. The second described his death over winter break. Just before Christmas, he had poured gasoline on himself in the bathroom of his family home.

Then he set himself on fire. The speculation online was that he had not done as well as expected in his first quarter at Stanford, and the shame had driven him to suicide.

Immediately, my mind went to what I could have done differently. I looked back at every email exchange I had with or about the student. There wasn't much. He had gone on academic leave near the end of the quarter, and I had granted him permission to take the final exam from home. But he didn't pursue this option, and in the rush of end-quarter finals and grading, I hadn't followed up. Rationally, I knew that not completing Intro to Psych was probably not the tipping point for this student. He may have suffered from depression or another mental illness. But whatever the reason for his death, I couldn't help feeling that I had treated a student's academic struggles too cavalierly. That some energy spent perfecting lectures would have been better put toward trying to connect with more students. If I had been more persistent in reaching out, I could have told him that lots of students struggle freshman year but go on to graduate with honors. He might have completed the course. Would that have made any difference? Maybe, maybe not.

Stanford doesn't make student suicides public, and I told only one trusted colleague and the graduate student who had been his TA in the course. Even though I didn't talk about the experience, the regret stayed with me—and remained my own private shame. Only years later, when I finally shared the story with a colleague who had become a close friend, did I realize how fundamentally the experience had shaped my approach to teaching. After that student's death, I dedicated myself to supporting struggling students. I made it my personal mission to help them understand that any single academic failure does not limit their future or define their abilities. (I remember telling more than a few freshmen about one of my favorite Stanford students, who got into medical school despite a transcript littered with C minuses and worse in his first two years. His letters of recommendation—including my own—raved about his perseverance and growth.) I adopted a policy of seeing every student as a human being first, before any discussion of grades or assignments. I tried to instill this philosophy in the teaching assistants I trained, and I made it the basis of every academic policy in the course.

To my surprise, I even found myself sharing this story in a recent workshop with community college faculty about finding meaning in education. When I thought about the most meaningful experiences of my teaching career, this was what came to mind first, despite the fact that I wish I could change history and stop it from happening.

What the University of Rochester program for physicians shows us is the importance of making time for these conversations. How we talk about stress matters. In most workplaces, families, and other communities, the way we talk about stress does little to support our well-being. We might complain casually about stress, reinforcing the fantasy of a stress-free life. Or we vent about our struggles instead of reflecting on what we can learn from them. Sometimes we choose to suffer in silence, preferring to avoid the vulnerability that comes with honest discussions about suffering. Hopefully, you have begun to pay attention to how you talk about stress as a way of practicing mindset mindfulness. Consider when and where there might be an opportunity to openly discuss the challenges you face, especially in the roles and relationships that are personally meaningful.

ONE OF my students, Patricia, was inspired by our class to have a conversation about stress with her daughter, Julie. Julie and her husband, Stephen, were fostering a one-year-old baby whose biological mother was homeless, addicted to drugs, and unable to care for the child. They had taken the baby home from the hospital and were ready to adopt. Instead, they had spent the last year waiting for the mother to give up parental rights. The waiting period had been full of visits from the biological mother and grandparents, as well as home inspections, trips to court, and meetings with social workers. Julie and Stephen felt like the baby's parents, but they had no idea if they would be able to raise the child.

Julie became so overwhelmed that she was thinking of asking her doctor for medication for depression. She felt completely beaten down and was starting to lose hope. From Patricia's point of view, Julie was strong and capable, exactly the kind of person who could handle such an agonizing process. Patricia decided to talk with Julie about stress mindsets, particularly the idea that Julie was up to the challenge she had chosen.

Together, they discussed how important this process was to Julie and her husband. They recalled the personal reasons that had made them want to be foster parents and their belief that someone needed to step up and be willing to go through this stressful process for the sake of the child. They talked about what had led to Julie and Stephen's decision to commit to this child in particular. Together, they found a point of view that put the year of stress into a bigger context.

Even though Julie and Stephen couldn't control the outcome, they knew they would rather stay the course than give up. So they began to take actions they could control, like joining a support group for foster parents and keeping up with all the necessary requirements to keep the adoption on track. The conversation Patricia and Julie had, and the positive changes it sparked, helped Julie so much that she no longer felt the need to begin taking antidepressants. I wish I could wrap this story up in a pretty bow and adoption papers, but at the time I write this, the process—both stressful and meaningful—is ongoing.

How you talk about stress with the people you care about matters. One way we know what we are capable of is through the eyes of others. When you take this view for them and with them, you help them see their own strength, and you remind them of the purpose of their struggles.

The Costs of Avoiding Stress

When we reflect on our daily lives, we might look back at a day that was very stressful and think, "Well, that wasn't my favorite day this week." When you're in the middle of one of those days, you might long for a day with less stress in it. But if you put a wider lens on your life and subtract *every* day that you have experienced as stressful, you won't find yourself with an ideal life. Instead, you'll find yourself also subtracting the experiences that have helped you grow, the challenges you are most proud of, and the relationships that define you. You may have spared yourself some discomfort, but you will also have robbed yourself of some meaning.

And yet, it's not at all uncommon to wish for a life without stress. While this is a natural desire, pursuing it comes at a heavy cost. In fact, many of the negative outcomes we associate with stress may actually be the consequence of trying to avoid it. Psychologists have found that trying to avoid stress leads to a significantly reduced sense of well-being, life satisfaction, and happiness. Avoiding stress can also be isolating. In a study of students at Doshisha University in Japan, the goal to avoid stress predicted a drop, over time, in their sense of connection and belonging. Having such a goal can even exhaust you. For example, researchers at the University of Zurich asked students about their goals, then tracked them for one month. Across two typically stressful periods—end-of-semester exams and the winter holidays—those with the strongest desire to avoid stress were the most likely to report declines in concentration, physical energy, and self-control.

One particularly impressive study conducted through the U.S. Department of Veterans Affairs, in Palo Alto, California, followed more than one thousand adults for ten years. At the beginning of the study, researchers asked the participants about how they dealt with stress. Those who reported trying to avoid stress were more likely to become depressed over the following decade. They also experienced increasing conflict at work and at home, and more negative outcomes, such as being fired or getting divorced. Importantly, avoiding stress predicted the increase in depression, conflict, and negative events above and beyond any symptoms or difficulties reported at the beginning of the study. Wherever a participant started in life, the tendency to avoid stress made things worse over the next decade.

Psychologists call this vicious cycle *stress generation*. It's the ironic consequence of trying to avoid stress: You end up creating more sources of stress while depleting the resources that should be supporting you. As the stress piles up, you become increasingly overwhelmed and isolated, and therefore even more likely to rely on avoidant coping strategies, like trying to steer clear of stressful situations or to escape your feelings with self-destructive distractions. The more firmly committed you are to avoiding stress, the more likely you are to find yourself in this downward spiral. As psychologists Richard Ryan, Veronika Huta, and Edward Deci write in *The Exploration of Happiness*, "The more directly one aims to maximize pleasure and avoid pain, the more likely one is to produce instead a life bereft of depth, meaning, and community."

Rethink Stress:
What Is the Cost of Avoiding Stress?

Although avoiding stress can seem like a rational strategy, it almost always backfires. One of the benefits of embracing stress is that you find the strength to pursue goals and endure experiences that are difficult but meaningful. The mindset exercise below will help you recognize the costs of trying to avoid stress in your life. Take a few minutes to write in response to any of the questions that seem relevant to your experiences.

1. Missed opportunities: What events, experiences, activities, roles, or other opportunities have you turned down or cut out of your life because you thought they were (or would be) too stressful?
   • Has your life been enhanced or narrowed by these choices?
   • What is the cost to you of missing these opportunities?

2. Avoidant coping: What activities, substances, or other "escapes" do you turn to when you want to avoid, get rid of, or numb thoughts and feelings related to the stress in your life?
   • Are these coping strategies a good use of your time, energy, and life? Do they enhance meaning or help you grow?
   • Are any of these coping strategies self-destructive?

3. Limiting your future: Is there anything you would like to do, experience, accept, or change, if only you were not afraid of the stress it might bring into your life?
   • How would your life be enhanced by pursuing any of these possibilities?
   • What is the cost to you of not allowing yourself to pursue them?

Final Thoughts

When psychologist Alia Crum—the triathlete who turned house-keepers into exercisers, and who now tries to change people's minds about stress—talks about her work to groups, she shares a story from her time as a graduate student. One night, she was working alone late in the basement of the Psychology Department at Yale, lost in a train of self-doubt, worrying about her research project and whether she would be able to finish it.

There was a knock on the door. The department's IT guy opened the door and looked in. Before Crum could say anything, he commented, "Just another cold, dark night on the side of Everest." Then he closed the door and walked away.

Two weeks later, Crum was lying awake in bed when his comment came back to her. "If you were climbing Everest, you can imagine it would be cold, and there'd be some nights it would be dark, and you'd be tired," Crum thought. "You'd be pretty miserable. But what did you expect? You're climbing Everest." At that time in her life, finishing her dissertation was her Mount Everest. She wasn't sure she would succeed. But that challenge was important enough to be worth weathering a few cold, dark nights.

Everyone has an Everest. Whether it's a climb you chose, or a circumstance you find yourself in, you're in the middle of an important journey. Can you imagine a climber scaling the wall of ice at Everest's Lhotse Face and saying, "This is such a hassle"? Or spending the first night in the mountain's "death zone" and thinking, "I don't need this stress"? The climber knows the context of his stress. It has personal meaning to him; he has chosen it. You are most liable to feel like a victim of the stress in your life when you forget the context the stress is unfolding in. "Just another cold, dark night on the side of Everest" is a way to remember the paradox of stress. The most meaningful challenges in your life will come with a few dark nights.

The biggest problem with trying to avoid stress is how it changes the way we view our lives, and ourselves. Anything in life that causes stress starts to look like a problem. If you experience stress at work, you think there's something wrong with your job. If you experience stress in your marriage, you think there's something wrong with your relationship. If you experience stress as a parent, you think there's something wrong with your parenting (or your kids). If trying to make a change is stressful, you think there's something wrong with your goal.

When you think life should be less stressful, feeling stressed can also seem like a sign that you are inadequate: If you were strong enough, smart enough, or good enough, then you wouldn't be stressed. Stress becomes a sign of personal failure rather than evidence that you are human. This kind of thinking explains, in part, why viewing stress as harmful increases the risk of depression. When you're in this mindset, you're more likely to feel overwhelmed and hopeless.

Choosing to see the connection between stress and meaning can free you from the nagging sense that there is something wrong with your life or that you are inadequate to the challenges you face. Even if not every frustrating moment feels full of purpose, stress and meaning are inextricably connected in the larger context of your life. When you take this view, life doesn't become less stressful, but it can become more meaningful.

Part 1 Reflections

Take a few moments to reflect on the questions below and consider sharing your **thoughts w**ith someone in your life.

1. How has your understanding of stress changed since you first picked up this book?
2. What lingering questions or concerns do you have about the idea of embracing stress?
3. What idea, study, or story from Part 1 stands out to you as most personally relevant and worth exploring in your own life?

PART 2

Transform
STRESS

What Does It Mean to Be Good at Stress?

IN 1975, SALVATORE MADDI, a psychologist at the University of Chicago, began to study the long-term impact of stress on employees at the Illinois Bell Telephone Company. It was supposed to be a simple longitudinal study. But in 1981, a cataclysm hit Bell Telephone. Congress passed the Telecommunications Competition and Deregulation Act, and the entire industry was disrupted. Within one year, Bell Telephone laid off half its workforce. Those who were left faced uncertainty, changing roles, and increased demands. As Maddi recalls, "One manager told me he had ten different supervisors in one year, and neither he nor they knew what they were supposed to do."

Some employees crashed and burned under the pressure, developing health problems and depression. Other employees thrived, finding a new sense of purpose and enhanced well-being. Because Maddi had been studying these employees for years, he had reams of psychological testing, personality profiles, interview notes, and other personal information. He and his colleagues began to search for clues in employees' files that could predict how they had responded to the stress.

A few things stood out about people who thrived under stress. First, they thought about stress differently. They saw it as a normal aspect of life, and they didn't believe that it was possible or even desirable to have an entirely comfortable, safe life. Instead, they viewed stress as an opportunity to grow. They were more likely to acknowledge their stress and less likely to view every struggle as a catastrophe headed toward a worst-case scenario. They believed that difficult times require staying engaged with life rather than giving up or isolating oneself. Finally, they also believed that no matter what the circumstances, they must continue making choices—ones that could change the situation or, if that wasn't possible, that could change how the situation affected them. People who held these attitudes were more likely to take action and to connect with others during stress. They were less likely to turn hostile or self-defensive. They were also more apt to take care of themselves, physically, emotionally, and spiritually. They built a reserve of strength that supported them in facing the challenges in their lives.

Maddi named this collection of attitudes and coping strategies "hardiness," which he defined as *the courage to grow from stress.*

Since that study of Bell Telephone employees, the benefits of hardiness have been documented across countless circumstances, including military deployment, immigration, living in poverty, battling cancer, and raising a child with autism, as well as in professions ranging from law enforcement and medicine to technology, education, and sports.

The benefits of hardiness can be observed even in extreme circumstances, and in parts of the world dealing with crises far greater than the economic disruption faced by Bell Telephone in the 1980s. Theresa Betancourt, a professor of child health and human rights at the Harvard School of Public Health, made her first trip to Sierra Leone in 2002. She was there to work with boys and girls who had been forced into war as child soldiers. Some of these children had been used as human shields and sex slaves. Others had been forced to kill family members or commit rape. "When people think of child soldiers, they think of people who are terribly damaged in some way," Betancourt said. "But I've seen very much the opposite: tremendous stories of resilience." Former child soldiers returned to school and dreamed of becoming doctors, journalists, and teachers. Public officials held cleansing ceremonies to help communities publicly forgive children and affirm their good nature. Families and communities came together to heal and move forward.

Betancourt has since conducted field studies in many regions where genocide, war, poverty, corruption, and AIDS have devastated communities. The consequences of such trauma are widespread and include stigma, guilt, shame, fear, depression, intrusive memories, and aggression. However, she has also witnessed strength, resourcefulness, and hope in survivors of the worst horrors imaginable. These seeds of resilience coexisted with the suffering.

In one of Betancourt's field studies, families in Rwanda were asked to describe what people in their community do to avoid hopelessness, worry, frustration, and deep sorrow. Several themes emerged from these interviews. Individuals who are resilient have *kwigirira ikizere*, sometimes referred to as a strong heart. They have self-confidence and courage in the face of challenges. Resilient individuals also show *kwihangana*, a trust in the future and in other people. They do not lose hope, and they find meaning in their problems. Resilience is also seen as a social process, not just an individual trait. The community must have *ubufasha abaturage batanga*—people come together in difficult times to support one another.

As these words from the Kinyarwanda language demonstrate,

the courage to grow from stress is universal. The strength to persevere, the instinct to connect with others, the ability to find hope and meaning in adversity—these are fundamental human capacities. They can emerge in times of stress no matter who you are or where you are.

SINCE SALVATORE MADDI first described hardiness in Bell Telephone employees, psychologists have gone on to coin many phrases to describe what it is to be good at stress: grit, learned optimism, post-traumatic growth, shift-and-persist, having a growth mindset. We've also learned so much more about how to cultivate these attitudes. But Maddi's definition of what it means to be good at stress—*the courage to grow from stress*—is still my favorite description of resilience. It reminds us that we cannot always control the stress in our lives, but we can choose our relationship to it. It acknowledges that embracing stress is an act of bravery, one that requires choosing meaning over avoiding discomfort.

This is what it means to be good at stress. It's not about being untouched by adversity or unruffled by difficulties. It's about allowing stress to awaken in you these core human strengths of courage, connection, and growth. Whether you are looking at resilience in overworked executives or war-torn communities, the same themes emerge. People who are good at stress allow themselves to be changed by the experience of stress. They maintain a basic sense of trust in themselves and a connection to something bigger than themselves. They also find ways to make meaning out of suffering. To be good at stress is not to avoid stress, but to play an active role in how stress transforms you.

The next part of this book will help you develop these qualities. We'll continue to look at the upside of stress, and the science that shows how stress can help you engage, connect, and grow. But more important, we'll look at how to get good at stress. We'll explore how to use the energy of stress, how to let stress be a catalyst for compassion, and how to find the upside in even the most difficult experiences. When you are able to do this, you transform stress from something to avoid into something to be harnessed.

engage | *how anxiety helps you rise to the challenge*

I MAGINE THAT YOU work for an organization with hundreds of employees and you're about to give a presentation to the entire group. The CEO and all the board members are in the audience. You've been anxious about this talk all week, and now your heart is pounding. Your palms are sweating. Your mouth feels dry.

What is the best thing to do in this moment: try to calm down, or try to feel excited?

When Harvard Business School professor Alison Wood Brooks asked hundreds of people this question, the responses were nearly unanimous: 91 percent thought the best advice was to try to calm down.

You've probably told yourself or others in moments of stress that if you don't calm down, you'll blow it. This is what most people believe. But is it true? Is trying to relax the best strategy for performing under pressure? Or is it better to embrace the anxiety?

Brooks designed an experiment to find out. She told some people who were about to give a speech to relax and calm their nerves by saying to themselves, "I am calm." Others were told to embrace the anxiety and say to themselves, "I am excited."

Neither strategy made the anxiety go away. Both groups still had nerves before their speech. However, the participants who had told themselves "I am excited" felt better able to handle the pressure. Despite feeling anxious, they were confident in their ability to give a good talk.

Feeling confident is one thing, but did they deliver? Yes. People who watched the speeches rated the excited speakers as more persuasive, confident, and competent than the participants who had tried to calm down. With one change in mindset, they had transformed their anxiety into energy that helped them perform under pressure.

Although most people believe that the best strategy under pressure is to relax, this chapter will reveal when and why the opposite is true. Whether it's a student facing the most important exam of her life or a professional athlete facing the toughest competition of his career, welcoming stress can boost confidence and improve performance. We'll look at how embracing your anxiety can help you rise to a challenge, and even transform a typical fear response into the biology of courage. We'll also consider strategies for turning threats into opportunities, and paralysis into action. Even in situations where you don't know what to do, how to do it, or if you can do it, embracing stress can help you find the strength to keep going. This chapter is an antidote to those times when stress makes you feel overwhelmed or powerless. When you stop resisting it, stress can fuel you. The strategies in this chapter will show you how.

Amped Up or Falling Apart?

If you were to enter the office of Jeremy Jamieson, a professor of psychology at the University of Rochester, the first thing you'd notice is a map of the United States that takes up an entire wall. The map labels every brewery in the country, even the most obscure microbrewers. As a connoisseur of beer, Jamieson says part of his mission as a professor is to turn students on to brews beyond Bud Light.

Jamieson played football as an undergraduate at Colby College, a small liberal arts school in Maine, and during his time as a college athlete, one thing struck him as curious. His teammates described their pre-game stress as being "amped up" and "excited." They even tried to increase their adrenaline, knowing it would help them perform. But when his teammates talked about the same adrenaline rush before exams, they used completely different language. Then it was "nerves," "anxiety," and "choking under pressure."

Jamieson wondered: Wasn't it actually the same thing? In both cases, stress was giving his teammates energy to perform. Why did they view stress as beneficial on the field but crippling before an exam?

That curiosity stayed with him as he went on to graduate school and began to conduct his own research. He started to suspect that people's fear of their own pre-performance jitters was rooted in negative beliefs about stress. "We're bombarded with information about how bad stress is," Jamieson says. But those beliefs don't reflect the fact that in many cases, our stress response truly helps us. Even in situations where it seems obvious that calming down would help, being amped up can improve performance under pressure. For example, middle school, high school, and college students who have greater increases in adrenaline during exams outperform their more chilled-out peers. Green Berets, Rangers, and Marines who have the highest increases in the stress hormone cortisol while undergoing hostile interrogation are less likely to provide the enemy with useful information. And in a training exercise, federal law enforcement officers who showed the greatest increases in heart rate during a hostage negotiation were the least likely to accidentally shoot the hostage. Despite most people's belief that some adrenaline improves performance, but too much impairs performance, the evidence suggests otherwise. When it comes to performing under pressure, being stressed is better than being relaxed.

Jamieson had a hunch that viewing stress as harmful interferes with people's ability to use stress as the resource that it actually is. If he could change people's minds about the effects of stress, he thought, he could help them use it to perform better under pressure.

Jamieson first tested his theory with college students preparing to take the Graduate Record Examination (GRE), an entrance exam for admission to PhD programs. He invited the students into a classroom to take a practice test. Before the test, he collected saliva samples from the students to get baseline measures of their stress response. He told all the students that the goal of the study was to examine how the physiological stress response affects performance. Then Jamieson gave half the students a brief pep talk to help them rethink their pre-exam nerves:

> People think that feeling anxious while taking a standardized test will make them do poorly. However, recent research suggests that stress doesn't hurt performance on these tests and can even help performance. People who feel anxious during a test might actually do better. This means that you shouldn't feel concerned if you do feel anxious while taking today's test. If you find yourself feeling anxious, simply remind yourself that your stress could be helping you do well.

Jamieson was hoping this message would boost students' performance. It worked. Students who received the mindset intervention scored higher on the practice exam than those in the control group. Importantly, there was no reason to believe that the difference in scores was based on differences in mathematical ability. Students had been randomly assigned to either receive the mindset condition or not, and the two groups also did not differ in SAT score or college GPA. Instead, it seemed as though embracing their anxiety helped students perform their best.

However, there was another possible explanation for the superior scores of those who received the pep talk. Jamieson's message about anxiety was awfully reassuring. What if instead of helping them use their stress, the message simply calmed them down? To test this possibility, Jamieson took a second saliva sample from students after the exam. If the intervention had calmed participants down, their levels of stress hormones should be lower than they were before the exam. If, on the other hand, the intervention had helped them take advantage of their nerves, their stress hormones should be as high, or even higher, than they were before the exam.

The proof was in the spit. The group that received the mindset message showed higher, not lower, levels of salivary alpha-amylase, a measure of sympathetic activation from stress. The message had not calmed the students down physically. In fact, they were more, not less, stressed. But most interesting was the relationship between stress and performance. A stronger physical stress response was associated with higher exam scores—*but only for students who received the mindset intervention*. The message had helped students take advantage of their stress and use it to fuel higher performance. In contrast, there was no relationship between stress hormones and performance in the control group. The stress response didn't help or hurt in any predictable way.

The mindset intervention changed the meaning of students' physical state in a way that changed its actual effect on performance. Choosing to see their stress as helpful made it so.

Over the next three months, the students took the real GRE and sent their scores to Jamieson's research team. The students also answered questions about how they felt during the test. The real exam had much higher stakes than the practice test. What would happen when the pressure was more intense?

Students who had received Jamieson's mindset intervention months earlier had a very different exam experience than students from the control group did. Although not necessarily less anxious during the exam, they were less worried about their anxiety. They felt more confident in their abilities and believed that their anxiety helped their performance. Most important, the students who had received the mindset intervention significantly outperformed the control students again. This time, the difference between groups was even larger than it had been on the practice exam.

IT'S WORTH taking a moment to ponder these findings. A few sentences spoken before a practice test months before students took the real GRE had an impact that could, conceivably, alter the path of their careers. This is what makes mindset interventions so exciting. When they work, they don't just have a onetime placebo effect. They stick. Jamieson didn't show up the day of the actual exam to remind the students to embrace their anxiety. He didn't need to. The message he had delivered was both true and helpful, and the students had somehow internalized it.

Mindset interventions don't just stick; they also snowball. Every time these students perform well despite—or perhaps because of—their nerves, they learn to trust themselves under pressure. If embracing anxiety changed students' experience of the GRE, how might it affect their performance on other exams? Or their confidence during graduate school interviews? Or even their ability to thrive in the pressure-cooker environment of graduate school?

Although Jamieson did not track these students after their GRE exams, other research hints at the broader impact of embracing anxiety. At the University of Lisbon, one hundred students kept daily diaries during an exam period. They reported how much anxiety they felt, as well as how they interpreted their anxiety. Students who viewed their anxiety as helpful, not harmful, reported less emotional exhaustion. They also did better on their exams and earned higher grades at the end of the term. Critically, the effects of mindset were strongest when anxiety levels were high. A positive mindset protected the most anxious students from emotional exhaustion and helped them succeed in their goals.

The researchers went a step further to see whether they could change students' experience of exhaustion after a stressful exam. They told some students who were about to take a hard test, "If you experience stress or anxiety, try to channel or use the energy those feelings may arouse in order to do your best." Another group of students was advised, "If you experience stress or anxiety, try to focus on the task to do your best." A final group of students was told simply, "Please try to do your best." After the test, students completed a measure of how depleted they felt by the experience. Those who had been encouraged to view their stress and anxiety as energy were the least exhausted.

A positive view of anxiety can also make you less likely to burn out in a demanding job. Researchers at Jacobs University in Bremen, Germany, followed mid-career teachers and physicians for one year to see if their attitudes toward anxiety influenced their well-being at work. At the beginning of the year, the teachers and doctors answered questions about their views on anxiety: Did they see it as helpful, giving them energy and motivation? Or did they view it as harmful? At the end of the year, teachers and doctors who saw their anxiety as helpful were less likely to be burned out, frustrated, or drained by their work. Once again, the effect of mindset was strongest for those who reported the highest levels of anxiety. The doctors and teachers who experienced the most anxiety were protected against burnout if they viewed anxiety as helpful. The researchers concluded that if people could learn to accept stress and anxiety as part of a challenging work life, that anxiety could actually become a resource rather than a drain on their energy.

Do you view anxiety as draining and depleting or as a source of energy? When nerves hit, do you interpret it as a sign that you aren't handling the pressure well, or do you interpret it as a sign that your body and brain are gearing up? Choosing to view anxiety as excitement, energy, or motivation can help you perform to your full potential.

Transform Stress: Turn Nerves into Excitement

As corny as it sounds, many of my students report that telling themselves that they are excited when they feel anxious really works. One of my students, Mariella, had recently become a yoga instructor—a dream job for her, but also one that triggered a lot of anxiety. She had all the physical signs of stress before every class that she taught. She had always labeled these sensations as "anxiety" and thought that her body's response was a problem. "I would worry that I was going to freak out and not be able to teach," she told me. "One time, I canceled a class five minutes before I was supposed to teach because I thought I was going to have a panic attack."

Mariella started to experiment with rethinking the physical signs of anxiety. "I still feel the same sensations, but I say to myself, 'This is good. This is my body trying to help me perform.'" Framing the pre-class nerves as excitement helped her channel the energy into her teaching. Rather than trying to manage her symptoms, she was able to turn her focus to her students and began enjoying teaching more.

Even though the familiar feelings of anxiety showed up before every class, she no longer needed to cancel class out of fear that she would have a meltdown and be unable to teach.

When you're anxious before a big event—be it a meeting, a speech, a competition, or an exam—remember that there is a fine line between anxiety and excitement. When researchers at the University of New Orleans strapped heart rate monitors onto experienced skydivers and nervous novices, they found that the more seasoned jumpers weren't calmer than those about to take their first leap. Instead, the experienced skydivers showed even higher heart rates before and during the jump. The more pumped they were to take the dive, the bigger their excite-and-delight response. When you need to take a leap and want to do well, don't worry about forcing yourself to relax. Instead, embrace the nerves, tell yourself you're excited, and know that your heart is in it.

Achieving the Dream: Putting the Science into Practice

The students in Aaron Altose's math class at Cuyahoga Community College in Ohio don't fit any one profile. Young single moms just out of high school sit next to middle-aged adults returning to finish a degree. Some students take three buses to get to class after work. Many have never seen an algebraic equation in their lives, but all of them need to pass this math course to fulfill a requirement. The other thing they have in common? Math anxiety.

Compared with only 25 percent of students at four-year colleges, 80 percent of students at community colleges report fearing math. This math anxiety can set off a vicious cycle. The anxiety makes students want to avoid math, so they skip class, ignore homework, and put off studying. The more they avoid math, the worse they do in class. This only reinforces their anxiety and convinces them they aren't good at math. The cycle of math anxiety, avoidance, and failure is a serious problem that contributes to low graduation rates at community colleges across the country. Fewer than 30 percent of community college students who are required to take a remedial math course ever pass, leaving more than 70 percent unable to complete their degree.

Altose is a dedicated teacher; his reviews on the website Rate My Professors include such praise as "Responds to emails more promptly than I do to my girlfriend." He left high school teaching to work at the community college level, where he feels better able to help his students make a real difference in their lives. He never thought he would end up teaching math. Like many of his own students, he had a terrible experience in his first college math course. "I didn't have a clue," he told me. "I thought, 'All these other people know math. If you're good at math, you can do this.' I liked math, but I couldn't do it. That made me think math wasn't for me." After a brief stint working at a hospital, Altose decided to go back to get a master's degree in math and teach the subject that had initially discouraged him.

At Cuyahoga Community College, Altose coached his math students on how to reduce their test anxiety. He gave them advice about stress management, lectured them about the importance of a good night's sleep, and even led relaxation exercises before exams. Nothing seemed to help. Then Altose met Jeremy Jamieson at an education conference in 2012. The event, sponsored by the Carnegie Foundation for the Advancement of Teaching, was designed to connect researchers with educators. Jamieson's counterintuitive stress mindset intervention intrigued Altose, and the two began a collaboration to test whether embracing stress would help Altose's community college students.

As part of a carefully conducted experiment, some of Altose's students received a stress mindset intervention just before their second math exam. The intervention explained how the stress response can improve performance, even when it's experienced as nerves, and encouraged them to view their anxiety as helpful rather than harmful during an exam.

So far, the results have shown that the mindset intervention is helping. Students are trying on the new view of stress, unprompted, like the student who told Altose one day, "Before a test, I feel bad, but maybe what I really feel is determined." Exam scores of the students who received the intervention improved, and end-of-semester grades went up.

There may be another lesson in these promising results. Like most teachers, coaches, and mentors, Altose had originally reinforced his students' beliefs that their anxiety was a problem. By emphasizing the importance of reducing stress before an exam, his advice only further confirmed what students feared: Anxiety was a sign that they would do poorly.

If you want to help people better cope with anxiety, a more useful strategy might be to simply tell them that you think they can handle it. Studies show that when people are told, "You're the kind of person whose performance improves under pressure," their actual performance improves by 33 percent. It doesn't matter whether the feedback is completely random. What matters is that the message changes the meaning of those first signs of anxiety. Instead of signaling "you're about to blow it," the nerves are proof that you're getting ready to excel. Telling people who are nervous that they need to calm down can convince them that they don't have what it takes. Trusting them to handle the pressure can help them rise to the challenge.

To Altose, if the stress mindset intervention helps students pass his course, it truly has the potential to change their lives. Cuyahoga Community College is an Achieving the Dream school, part of a national network dedicated to helping community college students complete their education. To many students, his math class is a major hurdle, a seemingly insurmountable barrier to achieving the dream. Passing the course is proof that the students' goals—a degree, a career, and their hopes for the future—are possible. Altose has seen the confidence that students have gained from conquering math translate to other courses, and then to other life goals.

THE ANXIETY-AVOIDANCE CYCLE Altose's math students can fall into isn't limited to academic stress. It shows up with every conceivable kind of anxiety, from phobias, panic attacks, and social anxiety to PTSD. The desire to avoid feeling anxious overtakes other goals. In the worst cases, people organize their lives around avoiding anything that provokes anxiety. And while they hope that this will make them feel safe, it tends to have the opposite effect. Avoiding what makes them anxious only reinforces their fears and increases their worrying about future anxiety.

I've had my own experience transforming the cycle of anxiety and avoidance. For years, a lifelong fear of flying kept me from getting on a plane. At first, I was willing to fly for important family events a couple of times a year. But then my fear got to be so strong that I would have a panic attack if I even thought about flying. My flight could be months in the future, and I would live with constant dread that whole time about the three hours I'd be airborne. So I made the choice not to fly. I really believed that the fear would go away if I knew I didn't have to fly.

After a few years, my decision began to feel like a self-imposed prison. I would have dreams about being in cities that I couldn't get to without flying, and then wake up anguished by the fact that I couldn't visit them. I worried that something would happen to a family member and I wouldn't be able to get on a plane. And the worst part? The feeling of being trapped by fear hadn't gone away. I was still trapped by fear; it had just turned its focus to the consequences of not flying.

Eventually I came to realize that I was paying the price of fear whether I flew or not. Avoiding flying had not, as I had hoped, gotten rid of my anxiety. So I made a conscious, terrified decision to choose to be afraid *and* to fly. I started small, with short flights. I hated every minute of it, but I valued being able to do it. I was able to attend events that I wanted to be at, like professional conferences, and those that I had feared I would miss, including my grandmother's funeral. Eventually, I came to realize that I preferred the meaning that flying adds to my life, over the illusion that I could prevent anxiety by avoiding the thing I was afraid of.

I wish I could say that I now love to fly. The truth is, I still dislike it, but I have gotten much better at it. Most important, I now fly several times a month, for work and to be with family. My first flight after years of refusing to board a plane was a short trip from San Francisco to Phoenix. Since then, I've flown throughout North America and to Asia and Europe. Every time I get on a plane, I feel both anxious and grateful to myself.

How to Transform a Threat into a Challenge

As we've seen, one of the most important ideas from the new science of stress is that we have more than one stress response in our repertoire. In a situation that requires us to perform under pressure—like an athletic competition, a public speech, or an exam—the ideal stress response is one that gives us energy, helps us focus, and encourages us to act: the challenge response. It gives us the motivation to approach the challenge head-on, and the mental and physical resources to succeed.

Sometimes, however, performance stress triggers a fight-or-flight response, the emergency instinct that has given stress a bad reputation. When a person has a fight-or-flight response under the pressure to perform, psychologists call this a *threat* response. A threat response isn't an overreaction of the stress response system—it's an entirely different kind of stress response, one that primes you more for self-defense than for success. Let's consider how these two responses differ and why the right kind of stress response can enhance your performance under pressure. We'll also look at what science can tell us about how to tap into a challenge response even when you feel threatened.

First off, there are important physiological differences between the two responses that can affect your immediate performance and the long-term consequences of stress. One of the biggest differences has to do with how stress affects your cardiovascular system. Both a threat response and a challenge response prepare you for action—something you can feel when your heart starts pounding faster. But during a threat response, the body is anticipating physical harm. To minimize the blood loss that might follow a nasty fight, your blood vessels constrict. The body also ramps up inflammation and mobilizes immune cells to prepare you to heal quickly.

In contrast, during a challenge response, your body responds more like how it does during physical exercise. Because you aren't anticipating harm, the body feels safe maximizing blood flow to give you the most possible energy. Unlike in a threat response, your blood vessels stay relaxed. Your heart also has a stronger beat—not just faster, but with greater force. Each time your heart contracts, it pumps out more blood. So, a challenge response gives you even more energy than a threat response.

These cardiovascular changes have implications for the long-term health consequences of stress. The kind of stress response associated with an increased risk of cardiovascular disease is a threat response, not a challenge response. The increased inflammation and blood pressure can be helpful in the short term of an emergency but can accelerate aging and disease when chronic. This does not seem to be true of the cardiovascular changes you experience during a challenge response, which put your body in a much healthier state.

In fact, the tendency to have a challenge response, rather than a threat response, is associated with superior aging, cardiovascular health, and brain health. Middle-aged and older men who have a challenge response to stress are less likely to be diagnosed with metabolic syndrome than those with a threat response. And in the Framingham Heart Study, one of the best-designed and longest-running epidemiological studies ever conducted in the United States, those with a challenge response physiology had a greater brain volume across their life spans. In other words, their brains shrunk less as they aged.

Your stress response also affects how well you perform under pressure. During a threat response, your emotions will likely include fear, anger, self-doubt, or shame. Because your primary goal is to protect yourself, you become more vigilant to signs that things are going poorly. This can create a vicious cycle in which your heightened attention to what's going wrong makes you even more fearful and self-doubting. In contrast, during a challenge response, you may feel a little anxious, but you also feel excited, energized, enthusiastic, and confident. Your primary goal is not to avoid harm, but rather to go after what you want. Your attention is more open and ready to engage with your environment, and you're prepared to put your resources to work.

Scientists have studied these different stress responses in many high-stakes situations, and a challenge response consistently predicts better performance under pressure. During business negotiations, a challenge response leads to more effective sharing and withholding of information, as well as smarter decision-making. Students with a challenge response score higher on exams, and athletes perform better in competitions. Surgeons show better focus and fine motor skills. When faced with engine failure during a flight simulation, pilots make better use of plane data and have safer landings.

These are just a few examples of scenarios in which a challenge response helps. Importantly, none of these studies showed that performance was enhanced by the *absence* of a stress response; it was enhanced by the presence of a challenge response. This is not a trivial distinction. If we think all stress responses sabotage success, we may rely on stress-reducing strategies that get in the way of peak performance.

Even what you learn from a stressful experience can differ depending on your stress response. A threat response is more likely to sensitize the brain to future threats. It will make you better able to detect threats and more reactive to similar stressful situations. The rewiring that takes place in the brain after a threat response tends to strengthen the connections between the areas of the brain that detect threats and trigger survival coping.

In contrast, when you have a challenge response, the brain is more likely to learn resilience from a stressful experience. In part, this is because you release more resilience-boosting hormones, including DHEA and nerve growth factor. The rewiring that takes place in your brain following a challenge response strengthens the connections between the parts of the brain's prefrontal cortex that suppress fear and enhance positive motivation during stress. In this way, a challenge response makes it more likely that you will experience stress inoculation as a result of your experience.

IS THIS A CHALLENGE OR A THREAT?

When you want to perform well, and aren't in danger, a challenge response is by far the most helpful stress response. It gives you more energy, improves performance, helps you learn from the experience, and is even healthier for you. But while a challenge response is ideal, a threat response is common in many situations that ask us to perform under pressure.

Psychologists found that the most important factor in determining your response to pressure is how you think about your ability to handle it. When faced with any stressful situation, you begin to evaluate both the situation and your resources. How hard is this going to be? Do I have the skills, the strength, and the courage? Is there anyone who could help me? This evaluation of demands and resources may not be conscious, but it's happening under the surface. As you weigh the demands of the situation against the resources you bring to it, you make a rapid assessment of your ability to cope.

This evaluation is the key to determining your stress response. If you believe that the demands of the situation exceed your resources, you will have a threat response. But if you believe you have the resources to succeed, you will have a challenge response.

Lots of studies show that people are more likely to have a challenge response if they focus on their resources. Some of the most effective strategies for this are acknowledging your personal strengths; thinking about how you have prepared for a particular challenge; remembering times in the past when you overcame similar challenges; imagining the support of your loved ones; and praying, or knowing that others are praying for you. These are all quick mindset shifts that can turn a threat into a challenge—which makes them good things to try the next time you want to perform well under pressure.

And yet, as it occurred to University of Rochester stress researcher Jeremy Jamieson, people often fail to realize one resource they have in every stressful situation: *their own stress response*. Because people view the stress response as harmful, it's considered a barrier to performing well. Then it becomes a burden to overcome. Jamieson, of course, has a very different view of the stress response's role in performance: It's not a barrier; it's a resource. If he could convince participants to see their stress response this way, could he not only boost their perceived resources but also change the nature of their stress response from threat to challenge?

Jamieson decided to conduct another study that would trigger a threat response in most participants without actually putting them in danger. For this, he turned to the Trier Social Stress Test, the most notorious and effective stress induction in human psychological research.

THE LABORATORY assistant brings you into a room and introduces you to a man and a woman seated behind a table. The assistant informs you that these two people are experts in communication and behavioral analysis. They will be assessing you today as you give a speech about your personal strengths and weaknesses. The experts will evaluate the content of your speech as well as your body language, voice, presence, and other nonverbal behaviors. "It's very important that you make a good impression," the assistant tells you. "Please do your best."

You've only had three minutes to prepare your speech, and you aren't allowed to use notes, so you're a little nervous. There's a microphone in the middle of the room. The assistant asks you to stand in front of the microphone to deliver your speech. She points a video camera at you and starts to record.

You smile and say hello to the experts. They nod but don't return the smile. "Please begin," one tells you. As you stumble your way through your speech, you notice some discouraging signs. One of the evaluators is frowning, staring at you with his arms crossed. The woman shakes her head disappointedly and scribbles something in her notebook. You try to increase your enthusiasm as you speak and try to make eye contact with the evaluators. The woman looks at her watch and sighs. Wait, did the man just roll his eyes?

These are the first few moments of the Trier Social Stress Test, or Social Stress Test for short. Ever since it was developed at the University of Trier, Germany, in the early 1990s, it has become the most reliable and widely used protocol for stressing out any human—male or female, young or old—in psychological experiments. And what you don't know is that these evaluators aren't experts at all. They've been hired to make you sweat. The experimenter has carefully trained them to make you as uncomfortable as possible. No matter how well you're doing, they will make you think that you're blowing it.

It starts simply enough, when you come into the lab and find out that you're going to have to give a speech to a panel of experts. Public speaking is one of the most common fears, so this makes most people uneasy. When you meet your evaluators they don't smile. If you make a joke, they don't laugh. If you express some nerves, they don't reassure you. As you give your speech, the evaluators begin to give discouraging nonverbal feedback. Standard instructions to evaluators in training include the following guidelines:

- Stare without emotion.
- Provide negative cues like shaking your head, furrowing your brow, sighing, rolling your eyes, crossing your arms, tapping your foot, frowning.
- Pretend to write things down.
- *No* smiling or nodding of the head or any other reinforcing behavior.

These "experts" are also encouraged to torment the participants in other ways. Some repeatedly interrupt to tell participants how poorly they are doing. One researcher told me that she instructs her evaluators to end every participant's speech by sighing heavily and saying, "Just stop."

I've been through the Social Stress Test, just to see what it was like. I thought I was fully prepared. I knew exactly what was going to happen, and when. I met my evaluators before the experiment began. We even joked about how stressful the experience would be.

It was even worse than I'd imagined. And I speak in public for a living.

The second part of the Social Stress Test is a timed math test. It's presented as a measure of your ability to think on your feet. You have to do the calculations in your head and answer out loud, as fast as you can. The math test, like the speech task and negative feedback, is carefully designed to stress participants out. One study found that when people anticipate having to do math, it activates areas of the brain associated with physical pain. The evaluators make the math test as miserable as possible. No matter how fast you go, they say you're going too slow. If you make a single mistake, you have to start the test all over. If you're doing well, they give you a harder task, to make sure you fail.

All this adds up to a thoroughly stressful experience. You have to perform under pressure, handle negative feedback, and navigate a confusing social interaction. All while doing two of the things that people fear most: public speaking and math. No wonder it's been shown to increase people's levels of the stress hormone cortisol by up to 400 percent.

This—the Social Stress Test, in all its glory—was the setup for Jeremy Jamieson's next mindset intervention study. Could rethinking stress transform how people responded to the most infamous stress induction in experimental psychology? Again, in particular, he was interested in whether rethinking stress could transform a threat response into a challenge response. For this study, he recruited women and men from the Harvard University community and throughout the Boston area via flyers and postings on Craigslist. They were invited, one at a time, to come to Harvard to participate in a psychology study. They had no idea what they were in for.

When each participant arrived, he or she was randomly assigned to one of three conditions. The first group got a mindset intervention. To help these participants rethink stress, Jamieson put together a few slides explaining how the body's stress response mobilizes energy to meet the demands of a situation. For example, when you feel your heart pounding, it's because your heart is working harder to deliver more oxygen to your body and brain. He also put together excerpts of scientific articles discussing how people commonly misinterpret their stress response as harmful, such as how many people believe that feeling anxious is proof that they lack the ability to do something or believe that the physical symptoms of stress mean they are going to choke under pressure. The last part of the intervention was an explicit mindset suggestion. Jamieson told participants, "When you feel anxious or stressed, think about how your stress response can actually be helpful."

Participants in the second group got a very different message about stress. They were told that the best way to reduce nerves and improve performance is to ignore stress. A few slides and articles hammered this point home for them—although, it should be said, these were phony articles and this is not great advice. They were a control group, and Jamieson did not expect the instructions to help them. Those in the third group got to blow off steam before the stress test by playing video games—they got no special stress instructions at all. After each participant went through whichever condition he or she had been assigned to—the mindset intervention, the instructions to ignore stress, or playing video games—the stress test began, and, with it, a test of Jamieson's hunch: that viewing your stress response as a resource can turn a threat into a challenge.

Let's get one finding out of the way: There were no differences in how those who were told to ignore stress or play video games performed in the social stress test. All the interesting effects were found in participants who had received the mindset intervention. For these participants, rethinking stress shifted their stress responses from threat to challenge in every conceivable way, starting with their perception of resources.

The mindset intervention had no effect on how difficult they expected the speech to be, or on how stressful they said they found the experience. However, compared with the two control groups, they felt more confident in their abilities to cope with the challenge.

Participants who received the mindset intervention also reacted to the stress test with a classic challenge response. Their hearts pumped out more blood with each heartbeat, and they did not show the degree of blood vessel constriction you would expect in a threat response. They also had higher levels of salivary alpha-amylase, a biomarker for stress arousal. They were more stressed, but in a good way. In contrast, the control groups showed the physiology of a typical threat response.

Each participant's speech was filmed. Afterward, Jamieson hired observers to analyze the videos. They noted each participant's body language, posture, and emotional expressions. They also rated the participants' overall performance. The observers didn't know which participants had received the mindset intervention, ensuring that their ratings would be unbiased. Participants who had gotten the mindset intervention were rated as being more confident and more effective overall. They made more eye contact with the evaluators, despite the eye-rolling they endured. Their body language was more open and confident—they smiled more, used more commanding hand gestures, and adopted the kind of expansive postures that psychologists refer to as "power poses." They also showed fewer signs of shame and anxiety, like fidgeting, touching their face, or looking down. The participants who had received the mindset intervention also made fewer self-handicapping statements, like apologizing for their nervousness. And, yes, they flat-out gave better speeches.

Jamieson went one step further to look at how the mindset intervention affected recovery from the stress test. After the math test, the evaluators left, and participants took a computer-based visual test of concentration. While the participants tried to focus on the test, the researchers attempted to distract them with words like *fear*, *danger*, and *failure*. Participants who received the mindset intervention were less likely to be distracted by these words and scored higher on the focus test. However stressful the stress test had been, they weren't letting it interfere with the next challenge.

Let's take a breath and appreciate the full scope of what the mindset intervention did. It boosted participants' perception of their resources to cope with stress. It shifted their cardiovascular stress responses from threat to challenge, without calming them down. They showed greater confidence and engagement, and less anxiety, shame, and avoidance. Objectively, they performed better. Afterward, they were less distracted by thoughts of fear and failure. And the catalyst for this transformation? One simple shift in how they thought about the stress response. The new mindset turned the body's stress response from a perceived barrier into a perceived resource, tipping the balance from "I can't handle this" to "I've got this."

Imagine how this mindset shift could add up over time. The difference between a chronic threat response and a chronic challenge response isn't just whether you can give a good speech or focus during an exam. It could mean the difference between feeling overwhelmed or feeling empowered by the stress in your life. It could even mean the difference between having a heart attack at fifty or living into your nineties.

Transform Stress: Turn a Threat into a Challenge

Viewing the stress response as a resource can transform the physiology of fear into the biology of courage. It can turn a threat into a challenge and can help you do your best under pressure. Even when the stress doesn't feel helpful—as in the case of anxiety—welcoming it can transform it into something that is helpful: more energy, more confidence, and a greater willingness to take action.

You can apply this strategy in your own life anytime you notice signs of stress. When you feel your heart pounding or your breath quickening, realize that it is your body's way of trying to give you more energy. If you notice tension in your body, remind yourself that the stress response gives you access to your strength. Sweaty palms? Remember what it felt like to go on your first date—palms sweat when you're close to something you want. If you have butterflies in your stomach, know that they are a sign of meaning. Your digestive tract is lined with hundreds of millions of nerve cells that respond to your thoughts and emotions. Butterflies are your gut's way of saying, "This matters." Let yourself remember why this particular moment matters to you.

Whatever the sensations of stress are, worry less about trying to make them go away, and focus more on what you are going to do with the energy, strength, and drive that stress gives you. Your body is providing you access to all your resources to help you rise to this challenge. Instead of taking a deep breath to calm down, take a deep breath to sense the energy that is available to you. Then put the energy to use, and ask yourself, "What action can I take, or what choice can I make, that is consistent with my goal in this moment?"

FROM "I WISH I DIDN'T HAVE TO DO THIS" TO "I CAN DO THIS"

One of my New Science of Stress students, Anita, was a graduate student studying neurological diseases. Throughout grad school, she had struggled with impostor syndrome. Anita wondered if she had what it took to be a researcher, and if she really belonged in the program. (As we've seen, this is a very common fear—but one that most people feel alone in.) Her qualifying exam, which would determine whether she would be allowed to continue in her PhD program, was scheduled for the week after our course ended. Every time she thought about her quals, she felt dread. She was convinced that she would fail spectacularly. She decided to use the class strategies to help her handle the pressure.

The lecture on seeing a stressful situation as a challenge versus as a threat was a major aha moment for Anita. She recognized all the elements of a threat response in how she was thinking about the exam. She felt like she didn't have the resources to cope, and she was convinced that her anxiety would cripple her during the test. She was avoiding the things that would help her prepare, like giving practice talks, because she wanted to avoid any feelings of anxiety and self-doubt. And even though the exam would get her closer to the career she had always dreamed of, she kept saying to herself, "I wish I didn't have to do this."

Anita decided to make a deliberate effort to shift her mindset from threat to challenge. She started with little things, like telling herself she was excited when she felt anxious, even though she didn't believe it at first. She reminded herself that her anxiety could actually be a resource, and that her body was giving her energy.

Then she started to change how she talked about the actions she needed to take—for example, meeting with each of her committee members. Anita was terrified that once she sat down and spoke with them about her project, they would realize that she didn't really know what she was talking about. She began to reframe the meetings as learning opportunities. She told herself, "Even if I don't know how to answer the questions they ask now, it will help me be better prepared for the exam." When she was less worried about not sounding stupid, she was better able to hear and make use of the feedback she received.

Anita also found the courage to give four practice talks. The first practice talk was to her lab group. She woke up that morning so nervous that she immediately thought, "I wish I didn't have to do this!" Then she caught herself and thought, "No, this will be useful. Even if my talk today is really rough and unpleasant to go through, I will learn from this experience, and my next talk will be better." Every time she gave a practice talk, she felt more confident and better prepared. When she told herself that she was adequate to the challenge, she found that she was starting to believe it.

By the time her quals date arrived, Anita woke up feeling like she might actually *be* excited. This was a big shock to her. She was still nervous before the exam, but for once in her life, she didn't worry about the anxiety. When she started her talk, her voice didn't waver like it usually did when she was nervous. And while she couldn't answer every question her committee asked, she maintained her composure and addressed them with confidence. At the end of the exam, her committee chair told her that it was the best presentation she had ever given.

Anita credits the turnaround to her mindset shift. "Realizing my anxiety was there, and that I shouldn't try to hide it or push it away or not feel it at all, was incredibly freeing. I didn't need to waste energy trying to *not* feel this way. I could just think about it in a different way."

Are There Limits to Embracing Anxiety?

One of the questions I often get is, "This whole 'embracing stress' thing only works if you don't have *real* anxiety, right?" Behind this question is a belief: Real anxiety is really, really bad. I really do need to get rid of it. If I embrace it, I'll fall apart. I need to fight it or it will consume me.

Well, there's something I haven't mentioned about Jeremy Jamieson's Social Stress Test study, the one that transformed threat responses into challenge responses. Half his participants had social anxiety disorder. The Social Stress Test was their worst nightmare.

Social anxiety disorder is a complex psychological condition, but one way to think of it is as a vicious cycle that traps people in social isolation. The cycle starts with anxiety about social interactions. People with social anxiety believe they are not good in social situations, so they worry about them in advance. They fear that they'll do something foolish and that others will judge them. They panic over whether they'll have to make small talk and be unable to escape. They might feel claustrophobic in groups and worry that they'll get stuck in a crowd.

When people with social anxiety disorder are actually in a social situation, they tend to focus on themselves instead of others. Thoughts run through their head: *I look stupid. Why did I just say that? Can they tell how nervous I am?* They feel awkward. They don't know what to say. As they grow more anxious, their sweaty palms and racing heart are taken as proof of their social inadequacy: *There's something wrong with me.* They start to worry that their anxiety is actually dangerous. *Why am I sweating so much? Am I having a heart attack?*

To cope, they engage in safety behaviors, like not making eye contact, staying in the bathroom too long, looking for a way out, going home early, or getting so drunk that they can't feel their own feet, let alone the anxiety. The self-focus and avoidance behaviors make it difficult to connect with others. So afterward, they think, "That was awful. I didn't do well at all. I guess I can't cope in social situations. Next time, I'll just skip the whole thing." It's a vicious cycle that feeds on itself. Eventually, the anxiety about social performance becomes anxiety about anxiety. It's a classic anxiety-avoidance cycle. Avoiding social situations becomes a strategy to avoid the anxiety—just like math anxiety can spiral into math avoidance, and my fear of flying kept me grounded and trapped.

The social situations that trigger social anxiety aren't just big events, with crowds and strangers. They can be a work meeting where you are expected to contribute a comment; or going to church, where you'll have to engage in small talk; or going to the store and having to ask for help. Social anxiety can affect very broad parts of a person's life. As the vicious cycle of anxiety and avoidance continues to spiral out of control, the world gets smaller and smaller.

Keep all this in mind, and then imagine what it would be like for someone with social anxiety disorder to go through the Social Stress Test. A student who helped Jamieson run the experiment told me that it was painful to watch. One woman started crying thirty seconds into her speech and didn't say anything else for the rest of the experiment. Another participant wrote on the post-experiment survey, "That was one of the worst experiences of my life."

The big surprise of the study was that embracing anxiety helped people with social anxiety disorder just as much as it helped people who didn't struggle with anxiety. In fact, the mindset intervention actually made those with the disorder look more like those without it. They were rated by observers as showing less anxiety and shame, and showing more eye contact and confident body language, than socially anxious participants who did not receive the mindset intervention. Their physical stress response shifted to a challenge response, and they had higher levels of the stress biomarker salivary alpha-amylase. And, just like participants who did not have an anxiety disorder, participants who had stronger stress responses were *more* confident, measured by both their own reports and observers' ratings. The mindset intervention did not calm them down; it changed the meaning, and then the consequences, of their anxiety. Think about this for a moment, especially if you have any experience with anxiety disorders or know someone who struggles with one: *Among people with an anxiety disorder who were encouraged to embrace their anxiety, a stronger physical stress response was associated with more confidence and better performance under pressure and social scrutiny.*

This is what shocks people the most. Even when anxiety really is a problem, embracing it helps. The value of rethinking stress is *not* limited to people who aren't really struggling. In fact, embracing the stress response may be even more important for those who suffer from anxiety. Here's why: Although people who have an anxiety disorder perceive their physiology as out of control, it actually isn't. In Jamieson's study, and in many others, people with anxiety self-report higher physical reactivity than those without anxiety. They think their hearts are pounding precariously fast and their adrenaline is surging to dangerous levels. But objectively, their cardiovascular and autonomic responses look just like those of the non-anxious. *Everyone* experiences an increase in heart rate and adrenaline. People with anxiety disorders perceive those changes differently. They may be more aware of the sensations of their heart beating or the changes in their breathing. And they make more negative assumptions about those sensations, fearing a panic attack. But their physical response is not fundamentally different.

When I joined the Stanford Psychophysiology Laboratory in 1999, one of my labmates had just finished running a study comparing the stress physiology of people with and without anxiety disorders. She found that they did not differ in stress physiology, even though the anxious participants perceived themselves as having stronger physical reactions. I remember so clearly sitting in the laboratory's data analysis room, working on my own set of physiological data, when my labmate shared her findings. I couldn't believe them. At the time, I struggled with anxiety, and I was convinced my own physiology was off the charts. I remember thinking that the lab must have failed to recruit people who were *really* anxious, since the findings made no sense. Of course, they make sense now that I know more about the role that mindset plays in changing the perception and consequences of stress arousal. But when I viewed my own anxiety as the enemy, I couldn't accept the findings.

Because people with anxiety have the most negative perception of stress, they are the most likely to be helped by a mindset intervention that teaches them to rethink the stress response. In my experience, they are also the least likely to believe it. I can fully appreciate this stance, having taken it myself. But I have also found that when it comes to mindset interventions, the more you initially resist the new idea, the more power it has to transform your experience of stress.

FROM WELFARE TO WORK

Sue Cotter recently retired from her job at the Community Services Agency in Modesto, California, to travel across the country in a camper van. For twenty-five years, Cotter had taught job readiness classes that helped welfare recipients find work. The classes took place at a sprawling complex that also included the office where people applied for food stamps, and the child welfare department where supervised visitations took place. Cotter knew firsthand what it was like to be in her students' situation. She had dropped out of school when she found out she was pregnant, and by age twenty-three, she had three kids and relied on food stamps. Although she eventually went back to school and earned her college degree in her thirties, she said that it took a lot for her to get to the point where that was even a possibility.

Cotter's students—who were all mandated to attend the three-week class—spent hours in her classroom drafting résumés, filling out online job applications, and practicing their interview skills. While these practical tasks made up the formal curriculum, Cotter's classes included an extra component. She conducted her own stress mindset intervention.

I met Cotter through a friend and was surprised to hear that she showed the video of my TED Talk on stress in her welfare-to-work classes. I was especially intrigued because one of the most frequent questions I get is whether rethinking stress is relevant for people living in extreme hardship. Cotter's students certainly seemed to fit the bill.

As Cotter described, most of the students who show up to welfare-to-work classes are one step away from being homeless. The assistance they receive—perhaps five hundred dollars a month for a single mom with one child—is not enough to pay rent and have a car. Some are in, or have recently left, abusive relationships. To attend the job readiness classes, they are forced to leave their kids in unreliable and potentially unsafe child care. Some have never held jobs. In recent years, the unemployment rate in Modesto has been as high as 20 percent, making their job search even more daunting.

Over the years she had taught job readiness classes, many of Cotter's student would go out and find a job, but then something would happen—they would lose their housing, get sick, or lose child care when a relationship broke up. Their lives fell apart, and they would end up back in class, trying to start over. "When you look at the number of things they have to deal with, just on a day-to-day basis, finding a way to deal with that stress is huge," Cotter said.

Soon after she began teaching welfare-to-work classes in the 1990s, she realized that the typical way stress management was taught wasn't enough. She had been trained to introduce the topic of stress by giving out a checklist of stressful life events. So Cotter gave her students the checklist and asked them to mark every one they had experienced in the past year. (I was taught to do this, too, as a health promotion strategy—and it's still a popular tool in stress-management trainings.) On the typical life-events checklist, each event is assigned a point value based on how stressful it is supposed to be. Getting divorced earns you seventy-three points. The death of a family member and spending time in jail are both worth sixty-three. Pregnancy gets a stress score of forty. Further down the scale, a change in living conditions merits twenty-three points, and surviving the holiday season earns twelve. When you add up your points, you get a stress score.

The point of the exercise? The higher your score, the more at risk you are for getting sick or dying. If you score in the highest category (three hundred points or more), the assessment you receive is simply, "You have a high or very high risk of becoming ill in the near future." As a stress-management tool, it's meant to shock people into realizing how important it is to do something about their stress. But imagine how it feels to check off half the things on the list—many of which you had no control over—and then be told that your life is so screwed up that it's going to kill you. One version of the scale I've seen includes the suggestion, "If you find that you are at a moderate or high level of risk, then an obvious first thing to do is to try to avoid future life crises." For many people—and certainly for Cotter's students—this kind of advice is laughable.

It didn't take Cotter long to scrap the life-events checklist after watching her students get discouraged by it. "It's depressing," she told me. "You realize, 'I might as well just give up, because I'm dealing with all this stuff, and I'll never get out of it.'"

As Cotter described her experiences to me, I thought of an email I had recently received from a psychologist who had seen me give a talk on embracing stress. He was very concerned about the message I was sending. "I fear the general gist people may get is that it's OK to live stressful lives and not do anything about it," he wrote.

I'm sure his concern comes from a genuine place of wanting to help. But when I read his email, the first thought I had was: What message does it send when we tell people it is *not* OK to live a stressful life? The truth is that most people don't choose the stress in their lives; they deal with it. When asked what is most stressful about their lives, people typically name things like a loved one's health problems, money worries, academic pressure, work stress, and parenting demands. We can't just excise these things from our lives to reduce stress. When people can't control what is stressful about their lives, how does it help to tell them that the reality of their lives is unacceptable?

Cotter had become convinced that the standard scare message about stress was exactly the opposite of what her students needed. "Everywhere you look," she told me, "you read about how stress causes all of these horrible diseases, and you think, 'I have no control over this life stuff that happens.' So how can it be that *that stuff* is going to control my future?" She saw over and over that the realities of her students' lives could paralyze them. Yes, they needed practical skills, stable living situations, and money—and Cotter tried to helped them get these things. But she also saw that they needed to believe there was something they could do in their lives that would make a difference—and many of them didn't.

So Cotter started to talk to her students about stress in a very different way. She explained that you can either let your stress overwhelm and paralyze you, or you can look at how to use that stress. She taught her students how a racing heart and fast breathing are your body's way of helping you cope with stress. "So when they're at that job interview and their hearts are pounding, they're not just thinking, 'Oh my God, I'm so overwhelmed,'" Cotter explained. They also talked about how to apply a challenge mindset when they faced unexpected stress. Cotter asked her students: What will you do when your car won't start on the way to work? How will you respond when the babysitter doesn't show up? She coached them through situations she knew they would face when they had a job, and she helped them plan in advance to take action rather than give up.

One thing that stands out about Cotter's students is they lack the kinds of resources that would help them easily handle situations like this. Many do not have a supportive family they can call on for help. They don't have money in the bank. In a way, the rethinking stress mindset intervention is perfect for them. The one resource they have is themselves. They have their own courage, their own persistence, and their own motivation. Viewing stress as a sign that things were out of control, and that they were falling apart, kept them from recognizing these strengths. "Rethinking stress empowers them," Cotter said. "It changes their beliefs about what they are capable of and what they can accomplish."

Cotter's observation reminded me of a little-known study I had stumbled across that was conducted at a domestic violence shelter in Colorado. In this study, researchers gave women a questionnaire that listed physical symptoms of anxiety, such as "Your heart is beating quickly," "Your palms are sweating," and "You feel short of breath." The questionnaire asked the women to imagine why they might be feeling this way. The options included neutral explanations like "You have been physically active," and positive explanations like "You are feeling excited." The survey also offered negative explanations such as "You're under stress and not handling things well" and "You can't deal with what's going on in your life."

The women who chose negative explanations for the physical sensations of anxiety perceived themselves to have fewer resources. They were more likely to blame themselves for the abuse, and they were at greater risk of developing both depression and post-traumatic stress disorder. They were also less confident about dealing with the legal system. The researchers' analyses showed that the women's tendency to interpret their physical sensations negatively was directly increasing these risks by making them doubt their coping resources.

This, I think, gets to the heart of what was happening in Jeremy Jamieson's studies, Aaron Altose's math classes, Sue Cotter's welfare-to-work trainings, and my own New Science of Stress course, when people decided to trust that their bodies' stress response could support them. Choosing to view a racing heart as a resource is more than a mindset trick that can transform your physical stress response from threat to challenge. It can also change how you feel about yourself and about your ability to handle what life is asking of you. Most important, it inspires action—and in this way, embracing anxiety helps you rise to the challenge.

Final Thoughts

I received a remarkable story via email that demonstrates how powerful embracing your body's response to stress can be. A woman was sitting on her back porch listening to my TED Talk on embracing stress. I had just finished explaining how the stress response can give you energy and courage. I described how a pounding heart was a sign that your body was rising to the challenge. At that moment, she heard a dispute in the house next door. She realized that a father was physically abusing his child. This was not the first time it had happened. Every time before, she had frozen. She had been abused herself as a child, and witnessing this abuse brought her back to her response to that trauma.

In the past, she had prayed for the child next door but had felt too paralyzed to act. This time, though, she took the TED Talk mindset intervention to heart. She thought, *My body can give me the courage to act*. And this time, she called the police. She marshaled her own inner resources and found the strength to call on outside resources for support. The police interviewed her and intervened to protect the child. In addition to helping a vulnerable child, she experienced her own capacity to break the cycle of fear and paralysis. And, to take it one step further, she shared the story with me, and now others—allowing her act to inspire others.

Is it always this simple? No. But stories like this are important reminders that the resources you need are already inside you. A shift in mindset and a leap of self-trust can help you harness them. The mindset reset this woman chose didn't change her history of abuse. It didn't take away her fear in that moment. But it did turn paralysis into courageous action.

Viewing your stress response as a resource works because it helps you believe "I can do this." This belief is important for ordinary stress, but it may be even more important during extraordinary stress. Knowing that you are adequate to the challenges in your life can mean the difference between hope or despair, persistence or defeat. Research shows that how you interpret your body's stress response plays a role in this belief, whether you are worried about an exam, getting over a divorce, or facing your next round of chemo.

Embracing stress is a radical act of self-trust: View yourself as capable and your body as a resource. You don't have to wait until you no longer have fear, stress, or anxiety to do what matters most. Stress doesn't have to be a sign to stop and give up on yourself. This kind of mindset shift is a catalyst, not a cure. It doesn't erase your suffering or make your problems disappear. But if you are willing to rethink your stress response, it may help you recognize your strength and access your courage.

connect | *how caring creates resilience*

I N THE LATE 1990s, two psychology researchers at UCLA were talking about how the female scientists in their lab responded differently to stress than the men did. The men would disappear into their offices, but the women would bring cookies to lab meetings and bond over coffee. Forget fight-or-flight, they joked. The women were tending and befriending.

The joke stuck in the mind of one of the women, postdoctoral researcher Laura Cousino Klein. Psychology research showed that stress leads to aggression, but that wasn't her experience. And it didn't fit with what she observed in other women either. They were more likely to want to talk with someone about their stress, spend time with their loved ones, or channel their stress into caring for others. She wondered if it was possible that science had neglected an important aspect of stress.

Klein decided to dig deeper into the science, and she made the surprising discovery that 90 percent of the published research on stress was conducted on males. This was true of animal studies as well as human studies. When Klein shared this observation with Shelley Taylor, the director of the lab she worked in, something clicked for her, too. Taylor challenged her lab to study the social side of stress, especially in women. Looking at both animal and human research, they found evidence that stress can increase caring, cooperation, and compassion. Under stress, women show an increase in tending—caring for others, be it their children, family, spouse, or other communities—and befriending, an increase in behaviors that strengthen social ties, such as listening, spending time together, and providing emotional support.

While the tend-and-befriend theory began as an investigation into the female response to stress, it quickly expanded to include men—in part because male scientists said, "Hey, we tend and befriend, too!" Taylor's team, along with other research groups, began to demonstrate that stress doesn't only motivate self-defense, as scientists had long believed. It can also unleash the instinct to protect your tribe. This instinct sometimes expresses itself differently in men than it does in women, but the two sexes share it. In times of stress, both men and women have been shown to become more trusting, generous, and willing to risk their own well-being to protect others.

When I was describing the tend-and-befriend theory in a recent lecture, a woman's hand shot up. "I think this theory needs a lot more analysis," she said. "This is completely contrary to my decades of experience in the business world."

I asked her to say more about that experience. "Stress makes people much more selfish," she declared, "protecting only themselves and undermining others."

This is a common reaction when people first hear about the tend-and-befriend response. My student wasn't wrong, exactly; she was describing one type of stress response. Stress doesn't always make us kinder—it can also make us angry and defensive. When the fight-or-flight survival instinct kicks in, we may become aggressive or withdrawn. Importantly, the tend-and-befriend theory doesn't say that stress *always* leads to caring. It simply says that stress can, and often does, make people more caring. Moreover, social connection is just as strong of a survival instinct as fighting or fleeing.

As we've seen before, how you think about stress plays a big role in determining what kind of stress response you have. We'll look at how to cultivate a tend-and-befriend mindset by focusing on bigger-than-self goals, supporting others, and even choosing to see stress and suffering as part of a common human experience.

Moreover, we'll find that the impulse to connect is both a natural response to stress and a source of resilience. When we care for others, it changes our biochemistry, activating systems of the brain that produce feelings of hope and courage. Helping others also protects against the harmful effects of even chronic or traumatic stress. In settings as seemingly disparate as a public transportation system challenged by rising crime rates, a "last hope" high school for poor and at-risk teens, and a prison hospital where inmates go to die, we'll see that caring creates resilience. Let's begin with a look at how a tend-and-befriend response helps you cope, and why choosing to connect with others makes you better at stress.

How Tending and Befriending Transform Stress

From an evolutionary point of view, we have the tend-and-befriend response in our repertoire first and foremost to make sure we protect our offspring. Think of a mama grizzly protecting her cubs, or a father pulling his son from the wreckage of a burning car. The most important thing they need is the willingness to act even when their own lives are at risk.

To make sure we have the courage to protect our loved ones, the tend-and-befriend response must counter our basic survival instinct to avoid harm. We need fearlessness in those moments, along with confidence that our actions can make a difference. If we think there's nothing we can do, we might give up. And if we are frozen in fear, our loved ones will perish.

At its core, the tend-and-befriend response is a biological state engineered to reduce fear and increase hope. The best way to understand how the tend-and-befriend response does this is to look at how it affects your brain. We've already seen that stress can increase levels of the neurohormone oxytocin, which activates our prosocial tendencies. But this is just one part of a tend-and-befriend response, which actually increases activity in three systems of your brain:

- The **social caregiving system** is regulated by oxytocin. When this system is activated, you feel more empathy, connection, and trust, as well as a stronger desire to bond or be close with others. This network also inhibits the fear centers of the brain, increasing your courage.
- The **reward system** releases the neurotransmitter dopamine. Activation of the reward system increases motivation while dampening fear. When your stress response includes a rush of dopamine, you feel optimistic about your ability to do something meaningful. Dopamine also primes the brain for physical action, making sure you don't freeze under pressure.
- The **attunement system** is driven by the neurotransmitter serotonin. When this system is activated, it enhances your perception, intuition, and self-control. This makes it easier to understand what is needed, and helps ensure that your actions have the biggest positive impact.

In other words, a tend-and-befriend response makes you social, brave, and smart. It provides both the courage and hope we need to propel us into action and the awareness to act skillfully.

Here's where things get interesting. A tend-and-befriend response may have evolved to help us protect offspring, but when you are in that state, your bravery translates to any challenge you face. And—this is the most important part—*anytime you choose to help others, you activate this state*. Caring for others triggers the biology of courage and creates hope.

A study by neuroscientists at UCLA demonstrated exactly how caring for others flips the brain's switch from fear to hope. The researchers invited participants to come to a brain imaging facility with a loved one. Once they arrived, the participants were told that this was a study about how people respond to others' pain. They were going to watch while their loved ones received a series of moderately painful electric shocks. To make sure the participants understood what their loved ones' pain would feel like, the researchers gave each participant a sample shock.

If they agreed to continue with the study, the participants wouldn't be able to prevent their loved ones from experiencing the pain, but the researchers did offer them two different ways to cope with the distress of knowing that their loved ones were suffering. During some of the painful shocks, participants were asked to hold their loved one's hands, to comfort them. During other shocks, participants were given a stress ball to squeeze, to help them manage their own stress about seeing their loved ones in pain. Throughout, the researchers watched what was happening in the participants' brains.

The two coping strategies participants used in this study—holding hands and squeezing a stress ball—are good examples of how we react to our loved ones' suffering in real life. Sometimes we turn our attention to our loved ones, to see if we can comfort, support, or help—

that's a tend-and-befriend response. It's an act of courage, even if all we do is listen and stay with them. Other times, we look for ways to escape the distress we feel about their suffering. This pulls our attention away from our loved ones and makes us less able or willing to help. We may retreat physically or mentally, turning to avoidance coping strategies to ease our own discomfort. Psychologists call this *compassion collapse*—by trying to avoid the stress we feel about *their* stress, we become paralyzed instead of mobilized.

The researchers in this study found that the two coping strategies had very different effects on the participants' brain activity. When the participants reached out to hold their loved ones' hands, activity increased in the reward and caregiving systems of the brain. Reaching out also decreased activity in the amygdala, a part of the brain known to trigger fear and avoidance. In contrast, squeezing the stress ball had no effect on the amygdala's activity. Like most avoidance strategies, squeezing the ball didn't reduce distress, and it actually *decreased* activity in the reward and caregiving systems—suggesting that it reinforced participants' feeling of powerlessness.

This study tells us two things. First, where we place our attention when people we care about are suffering can change our own stress response. If we focus on comforting, helping, and caring for our loved ones, we experience hope and connection. If, instead, we focus on relieving our own distress, we stay stuck in fear. The second thing this study shows is that we can create the biology of courage through small actions. In this case, it was holding a loved one's hand while he or she experienced pain. In everyday life, there are many opportunities to make similar small choices of connection.

Whether you are overwhelmed by your own stress or the suffering of others, the way to find hope is to connect, not to escape. The benefits of taking a tend-and-befriend approach go beyond helping your loved ones, although this, of course, is an important function. In any situation where you feel powerless, doing something to support others can help you sustain your motivation and optimism.

THIS SIDE effect of a tend-and-befriend response makes helping others a surprisingly effective way to transform stress. For example, researchers at the Wharton School of the University of Pennsylvania were interested in finding a way to relieve time pressure at work. You know the feeling: There's too much to do and not enough time to do it. Time scarcity is not just a stressful feeling; it's a state of mind that has been shown to lead to poor decisions and unhealthy choices. In this study, the Wharton researchers tried out two different ways to relieve the feeling of not having enough time. They gave some people an unexpected windfall of free time and asked them to spend it however they wished. Others were asked to spend that time helping someone else. Afterward, the researchers asked participants to rate both how much free time they had available right now and how scarce a resource time was for them in general.

Surprisingly, helping someone else decreased people's feeling of time scarcity more than actually giving them extra time did. Those who had helped someone else reported afterward that they felt more capable, competent, and useful than people who had spent the time on themselves. This, in turn, changed how they felt about what they had to accomplish and their ability to handle the pressure. In this way, the experiment resembles Jeremy Jamieson's embrace-mindset interventions—helping others boosted their self-confidence, which changed how they felt about the demands they faced. Their newfound confidence also changed how they perceived something as objective as time; after helping someone else, time, as a resource, expanded.

From a tend-and-befriend point of view, we might speculate that helping others shifted their biology, dampening their feelings of overwhelm. The Wharton researchers summarized their findings with this advice: "When individuals feel time constrained, they should become more generous with their time—despite their inclination to be less so."

This advice is spot-on, not least because people often underestimate how good they will feel when they help others. For example, people wrongly predict that spending money on themselves will make them happier than spending money on others, when the reverse is true. Giving can boost your mood even when you are forced to do it. In one study, economists at the University of Oregon gave all participants one hundred dollars and then asked them if they wanted to donate some of the money to a local food bank. Pretty much everyone gave something, though participants' altruism varied. The researchers also took some money back without the participant's consent and donated it to the food bank in the participant's name. In both situations, and among most participants, the brain's reward system became activated by the donations. The brain changes were stronger when participants chose to make the donation themselves, but in both scenarios, the direction of change was the same. Those brain changes also predicted a boost in mood—giving to the food bank made most participants feel good.

The takeaway of these two studies isn't that people should be forced to be more charitable or to help others. Rather, these findings remind us that we don't necessarily need to wait until we feel uplifted by a sense of generosity to decide to help someone out. Sometimes, we make the choice to be generous first, and the uplift comes later. Especially when you are feeling like your own resources—whether time, energy, or otherwise—are scarce, choosing to be generous is a way to access the resilience that goes along with a tend-and-befriend response. If you struggle with avoidance, self-doubt, or feeling overwhelmed, helping others is one of the most powerful motivation boosters that you can find.

Transform Stress: Turn Overwhelmed into Hopeful

When you are feeling overwhelmed, look for a way to do something for someone else that goes beyond your daily responsibilities. Your brain might tell you that you don't have the time or energy, but that is exactly why you should do it. You can also make this a daily practice—set a goal of finding an opportunity to support someone else. By doing so, you prime your body and brain to take positive action and to experience courage, hope, and connection.

Two strategies can amplify the benefit of this practice. First, your brain's reward system will get a bigger boost from doing something new or unexpected than if you do the same kind act every day. Second, small acts can be just as powerful as grand gestures, so look for little things you can do instead of waiting for the perfect moment to be magnanimous. I encourage my students to be creative in what they decide to be generous with. You can give others appreciation, your full attention, or even the benefit of the doubt. Like other mindset resets we've seen—such as remembering your values or rethinking your racing heart—it's a small choice that can have unexpectedly large effects on how you experience stress.

How Bigger-Than-Self Goals Transform Stress

During the 1999–2000 academic year, psychology researcher Jennifer Crocker was on a sabbatical, taking a break from her teaching and administrative duties at the University of Michigan. Although sabbaticals are often idealized as a time to restore creative energies and devote oneself more fully to research, the truth is that Crocker was just plain burned out. She had taken a professorship at the University of Michigan a few years earlier. The school had one of the top psychology research programs in the world, and many of her colleagues were famous in the field. Despite being selected for her own outstanding research—poached, in fact, from another prestigious school—she continued to wonder whether the hiring committee had made a mistake, and if she really was what her colleagues referred to as "Michigan material." (As a side note, I have to say how surprised I was to hear Crocker say this. Her CV includes over a hundred scientific publications and a dozen major awards, including a Distinguished Lifetime Career Award that was granted in 2008.) After several years of trying to prove her worth, she was drained and exhausted. Now she was taking time off to figure out how to reengage with her goals without running herself into the ground.

During the spring of her sabbatical year, Crocker had coffee with a good friend who urged her to attend a professional leadership workshop in Sausalito, California. Crocker gave in, not expecting much. Instead, what she heard during the nine-day workshop was exactly what she needed. It focused on the costs of being driven to prove your worth, just as Crocker had experienced. Fellow participants in the workshop included executives, physicians, and even parents with their teenagers—and Crocker was surprised to find that every single person in the room seemed to relate to this message as well. It was exhausting to approach the goals in your life from a place of constant competition, always trying to impress others or prove yourself. It drained the joy out of work. It created conflict in relationships. It took a toll on health. And yet everyone there, like Crocker, thought this was the only way to succeed.

The workshop leaders, however, had a different point of view. They argued that if you see yourself as part of something bigger—a team, an organization, a community, or a mission—it takes the toxicity out of striving. When your primary goal is to contribute to this "something bigger," you still work just as hard, but the motivation driving you is different. Rather than just trying to prove that you are good enough or better than others, you view your efforts as serving a purpose greater than yourself. Instead of focusing on only your own success, you also want to support others to further the broader mission.

The participants, including Crocker, were encouraged to contemplate their bigger-than-self goals, defined as a purpose that goes beyond the goals of personal gain and success. A bigger-than-self goal is not an objective goal, like getting a promotion, or a reward, like being praised by your boss. It is more about how you see your role within your community—what you want to contribute, and the change you want to create. When you strive from this mindset, the workshop leaders explained, you increase your chance of reaching both your professional and bigger-than-self goals—and you also experience more joy and meaning along the way.

Crocker realized that for her entire professional life, she had been driven from a mindset of competition and self-focus, rather than a bigger-than-self goal. Learning a new way to approach her work seemed like a radical but exciting solution to the burnout she had experienced. But Crocker was still a scientist first. So when her sabbatical ended, she did what any good researcher would do: She started designing studies to find out how these two different mindsets work.

CROCKER AND her colleagues have studied the consequences of self-focused versus bigger-than-self goals for academic success, workplace stress, personal relationships, and well-being, as well as in two very different cultures, the United States and Japan. One of the first things they found is that when people are connected to bigger-than-self goals, they feel better: more hopeful, curious, caring, grateful, inspired, and excited. In contrast, when people are operating from self-focused goals, they are more likely to feel confused, anxious, angry, envious, and lonely.

The emotional consequences of these goals build up over time, so people who persistently pursue self-focused goals are more likely to become depressed, while those who pursue bigger-than-self goals show greater well-being and satisfaction with their lives. One reason for this difference is that people who operate from a bigger-than-self mindset end up building strong social support networks. Paradoxically, by focusing on helping others instead of proving themselves, they become more respected and better liked than people who spend more energy trying to impress others than they do supporting them. In contrast, people who relentlessly pursue self-focused goals are more likely to be resented and rejected by others, and to experience a decline in social support over time. Like Crocker before her sabbatical, they may succeed professionally but still feel isolated and insecure about their standing.

Importantly, these two ways of pursuing goals are not fixed personality traits. Crocker has shown that everyone has both types of goals—to prove themselves and to contribute to something bigger than themselves—and that these motivations fluctuate over time. (One primary factor seems to be the people around us; Crocker has found that both self-focused and bigger-than-self goals are contagious.) In her earliest experiments, she tried to manipulate people's motivations with all kinds of psychological tricks, including priming different goals outside participants' conscious awareness. But she soon realized that it works much better when people have to make the shift themselves. When people are invited to reflect on their bigger-than-self goals, they can switch mindsets. Moreover, when they do, it transforms their experience of stress.

In one study, Crocker and her colleagues tested the effects of thinking about bigger-than-self goals on how participants experience a stressful job interview. Some participants were given a brief mindset intervention before the interview. The experimenter explained that job interviews tend to put people in a competitive and self-promoting state of mind. Another way to approach an interview, the experimenter suggested, is to focus on how getting the job would allow you to help others, or contribute to a larger mission. Instead of trying to prove yourself, you could focus on something bigger than yourself. Participants were given a couple of minutes to think about their most important values, and how the job would allow them to help others and make a difference. Most notably, the experimenter didn't impose any bigger-than-self goals; participants had to find them for themselves.

To examine how the mindset shift affected performance, the study measured participants' stress hormones before and after the job interview. They also videotaped the interviews and hired unbiased observers to analyze the participants' behavior. Participants who had reflected on their bigger-than-self goals showed more signs of affiliation with the interviewers, such as smiling, making eye contact, and unconsciously mimicking the interviewers' body language—all behaviors shown to increase rapport and strengthen social connection. Further, raters preferred what these participants had to say, rating their answers as more inspiring than the responses of participants who had not contemplated their values. The mindset shift also influenced participants' physical stress responses. Those who had reflected on their bigger-than-self goals for the job showed less of a threat response, as measured by two stress hormones, cortisol and adrenocorticotropic hormone (ACTH).

Crocker isn't the only researcher who has investigated the benefits of taking a tend-and-befriend approach to achieving personal goals. David Yeager, whom we met in Chapter 1 (when he was delivering a growth mindset intervention to ninth graders in gym shorts), has shown that helping students find their bigger-than-self goals improves academic motivation and performance. In one study, college students were given a twenty-minute "beyond-the-self" mindset intervention that included this exercise:

> Take a moment to think about what kind of person you want to be in the future. Also think about what kind of positive impact you want to have on the people around you or society in general. . . . In the space below, write a few sentences that answer this question: How will learning in school help you be the kind of person you want to be, or help you make the kind of impact you want on the people around you or society in general?

Students were then given a series of both boring and difficult math problems. The students who had completed the beyond-the-self reflection persisted longer and ended up finishing more problems correctly. The same brief mindset intervention in high school students not only boosted short-term motivation, but also led to higher end-of-semester GPAs. Yeager and his colleagues found that when students thought about their bigger-than-self goals, it changed the meaning of both boring work and academic struggles. The new meaning—that persevering at their studies would help them make a difference in the world—motivated them to engage with, rather than avoid, the stress of challenging themselves.

A study at Case Western Reserve University provides more insight into why bigger-than-self goals transform stress so effectively. In this study, neuroscientists brought students into the lab to have a conversation with an academic advisor. For some of the participants, the advisors took a straightforward approach to the meeting, diving into the usual discussion about students' work and any problems they faced. With other participants, the advisor asked about the student's vision for his or her future, prompting a reflection on their values and ideals. All the while, the neuroscientists tracked the activity in each student's brain. When the advisor asked about students' bigger-than-self purpose, the students felt more inspired, cared for, and hopeful. It also increased activity in all three brain systems associated with a tend-and-befriend response to stress. Reflecting on your bigger-than-self goals seems to have the same effect as helping others; it harnesses the positive motivation that comes with a tend-and-befriend response.

Transform Stress: Turn Self-Focus into Bigger-Than-Self Goals

When you feel stress rising at work or in any other important area of your life, ask yourself, "What are my bigger-than-self goals?" and "How is this an opportunity to serve them?"

If you're struggling to find a bigger-than-self goal, consider spending a few moments reflecting on one or more of these questions:

- What kind of positive impact do you want to have on the people around you?
- What mission in life or at work most inspires you?
- What do you want to contribute to the world?
- What change do you want to create?

Designing Bigger-Than-Self Goals into the Workplace

Monica Worline is a founding member of the CompassionLab Research Group, a collective of organizational psychologists who study social connection in the workplace. Her research shows that feeling connected to others in the workplace decreases burnout and increases employee engagement—with the biggest benefits coming from being able to help others.

As president of her own consulting company based in San Diego, Worline has worked with twenty companies on the NASDAQ-100 index, as well as many on *Fortune* magazine's list of "World's Most Admired Companies." One exercise she uses to help businesses increase employee resilience is called *role redesign*—rewriting your job description from a bigger-than-self perspective. Most job descriptions list the tasks involved, the skills required, and the priorities of the position. But they rarely give you a sense of the *why*—the contribution the person in the job makes to the organization or the community.

In role redesign, Worline asks people to consider: What if you described your job from the point of view of the people you work with or serve? What would they say about how your role helps them? How does your job support the greater mission of the company or the welfare of people in your community? Although this reframing doesn't change the basic tasks of the job, it does shift how people perceive them. Worline has found that this exercise reliably increases the meaning and satisfaction people take from their work.

One of her favorite examples of designing bigger-than-self goals into the workplace happened in Louisville, Kentucky, at a time when there were growing concerns about safety on the public transit system. For example, in July 2012, the city was shocked when three men got into an argument at the back of a bus, and one pulled out a gun and killed seventeen-year-old Rico Robinson in broad daylight. Louisville mayor Greg Fischer challenged the transportation system to increase public safety. Part of the initiative included asking the city bus drivers to consider how they could play a role in protecting the well-being of their passengers, beyond the already-installed security cameras and emergency radios.

The bus drivers took the challenge seriously and collectively renamed themselves "safety ambassadors." Driving the bus was still their primary task, but they began to reimagine their role to include making the bus a space where passengers felt seen and known. They decided that one thing they could do was greet passengers when they boarded the bus. Not just take their money or check their passes, but also make eye contact and say hello. By connecting with every passenger, the bus drivers could reduce the anonymity that encourages crime in public spaces. They could make their riders feel more comfortable and welcomed.

The biggest surprise of the role redesign was how it affected the bus drivers. Their sense of the meaning of their work went through the roof, Worline said—an especially important outcome in a job that has a high risk of burnout. (According to *U.S. News and World Report*, bus drivers face above-average stress levels but below-average opportunities for advancement.) For the Louisville bus drivers, reimagining themselves as safety ambassadors changed the meaning of their jobs. They were serving the bigger-than-self purpose of supporting the mayor's safety initiative in their community—and they got to connect to this goal every time someone boarded their bus.

Worline says that the Louisville case echoes her experience with every group she's ever worked with. When you see your job through a bigger-than-self mindset, it can elevate even the most basic tasks, and buffer against burnout.

THE BENEFITS of bigger-than-self goals are not limited to job satisfaction. Research also shows that leaders who apply this mindset to key decisions can help their organizations rebound from adversity. In 2013, researchers at the University of Virginia and the University of Washington surveyed the leadership of 140 companies that had gone through a major hardship in the past two years. The companies represented many industries, including manufacturing, service, retail, and agriculture. In addition to struggling with a prolonged economic recession, all had dealt with at least one serious threat to their company's future.

The researchers interviewed the leaders to find out what they had done to survive during that time. They also looked at the companies' financial reports to see how the crisis affected revenues, profits, and organizational size. When the researchers compared the companies that thrived with those that suffered the most, one key difference jumped out: The most successful companies had taken what the researchers called a collectivistic approach to dealing with hardship. In other words, they used the crisis as an opportunity to support something bigger than themselves. For example, several companies had struggled with local crime. Most responded by installing extra security and trying to strengthen the barriers between their company and the immediate neighborhood environment. One business, however, tried an unusual tend-and-befriend strategy: It invested in and restored nearby abandoned buildings, then rented them out to the community.

Some of the other effective and creative bigger-than-self solutions that companies reported included responding to a recession by offering discounts to important community groups, such as police officers and schools, and addressing a shortage of skilled workers by creating a mentoring and scholarship program for local youths. In each of these cases, the company's leaders decided to focus on the greater community good, and not only their own immediate survival. Importantly, these weren't just feel-good solutions. Across industries, when leaders sought bigger-than-self solutions, the companies showed greater revenue growth, profits, and expansion during and after the crisis.

Many people mistakenly assume that compassion is a weakness and that caring about others will deplete our resources. But what the science and these examples show is that caring can actually amplify our resources. Because social species—including human beings—cannot survive on their own, nature has equipped us with an entire motivational system that ensures we care for one another. In many ways, this system is even more crucial to our survival than the fight-or-flight instinct. Perhaps that is why nature bestowed it with the power to give us not just energy but also hope, courage, and even intuition. When we engage that motivational system through tending and befriending, we also tap into the resources we need to handle our own challenges and make wise decisions. Far from being a drain, tending and befriending can empower us.

How Caring Creates Resilience

Natalie Stavas, a thirty-two-year-old physician, was nearing the end of the Boston Marathon, having just run twenty-six miles on a broken foot. She was determined not to let the injury keep her from raising money for the children's hospital where she worked. As she neared the finish line, Stavas heard what she thought were fireworks. Then came the swarm of people screaming and running toward her.

It was April 15, 2013. The unthinkable had happened.

Stavas turned to her father, who had been running the marathon alongside her, and said, "Dad, we have to get there to help." She jumped a four-foot race barricade and took off down an alley. She soon found herself outside the Atlantic Fish Co., the scene of the second bomb's explosion. Blood was everywhere—so thick in the air that she could literally taste it. Stavas tried to get her bearings as she surveyed the scene. An abandoned stroller. A foot with no body. Then she saw a young woman lying on the ground. She checked for a pulse and began pumping the woman's chest.

Stavas treated five people at the scene of the explosion. Four survived. She didn't stop trying to help until a cop dragged her away.

Stavas was one of the many who rushed into action after the bombs went off. Runners who had just finished the marathon raced to Massachusetts General Hospital to give blood. Online platforms for "crowd-caring" popped up, where locals offered stranded runners food, company, and places to sleep. Volunteers returned to the finish line to retrieve the race medals and belongings that terrified runners had left behind.

These acts of caring didn't happen days or weeks later, as people struggled to make sense of a tragedy. The urge to do something was instinctive.

The outpouring of help that took place in Boston is touching, but not extraordinary. Its very ordinariness is the point: Difficult circumstances give rise to great acts of kindness because suffering provokes a basic need to help others. Studies show that after any sort of traumatic event, most people become more altruistic. They spend more time caring for friends and family, as well as volunteering for nonprofit organizations and church groups. Importantly, this altruism helps them cope. The more time trauma survivors spend helping others, the happier they are and the more meaning they see in their lives.

The instinct to help others when you, yourself, are struggling has been dubbed "altruism born of suffering" by Ervin Staub, a professor of psychology at University of Massachusetts, Amherst. In his youth, Staub escaped Nazism and Communism in Hungary. As a researcher, he had intended to study the conditions that lead to violence and dehumanization, but along the way, he became fascinated by the stories of helping that kept surfacing—such as the 82 percent of Holocaust survivors who said they went out of their way to help others while they were imprisoned, sharing the little food that they had even while starving.

Staub has documented an increase in altruism in the aftermath of community-wide traumas such as natural disasters, terrorist attacks, and war, and one thing stands out about altruism after such tragedies: People who have suffered the most also help the most. After Hurricane Hugo struck the southeast United States in 1989, people who were hit the worst provided more help to other victims than locals who were less affected by the storm. After 9/11, Americans who reported the most distress also donated the most time and money to support victims of the attacks. More broadly, Staub has found that people who have suffered a high number of traumatic events in their lives are more likely to volunteer or donate money after natural disasters.

This can seem a puzzling phenomenon if you view altruism as a drain on your own resources. From this point of view, our own losses should motivate us to conserve energy and hold on to whatever resources we have left. Why would suffering make people so eager to be of service?

The answer seems to lie in something we've already considered: how caring creates courage and hope. As we've seen, helping others can transform fear into bravery, and powerlessness into optimism. When life is most stressful, this benefit of tending and befriending is even more crucial to our survival. The instinct to help when we, ourselves, are struggling plays an important role in preventing a *defeat response*. The defeat response is a biologically hardwired response to repeated victimization that leads to loss of appetite, social isolation, depression, and even suicide. Its main effect is to make you withdraw. You lose motivation, hope, and the desire to connect with others. It becomes impossible to see meaning in your life, or to imagine any action you could take that would improve the situation. Not every loss or trauma leads to a defeat response—it kicks in only when you feel that you have been beaten by your circumstances or rejected by your community. In other words, when you think there is nothing left that you can do and nobody who cares. As awful as it sounds, a defeat response is nature's way of removing you from the picture so you don't use up communal resources.

Like the fight-or-flight and tend-and-befriend responses, the defeat response is found in every social species. And yet a defeat response, from an evolutionary point of view, should be an absolute last resort. Therefore, we need a counter instinct that can kick in when we start to despair, to keep us engaged with life even when things seem hopeless. That instinct is the tend-and-befriend response or, as Ervin Staub calls it, altruism born of suffering. When you help someone else in the middle of your own distress, you counter the downward spiral of defeat. As one woman who served food to rescue workers at the World Trade Center after the 9/11 terrorist attacks said, "I am proud to be able to have done something. . . . But it was this weird thing, like you were just desperate to do something and it was also about you as much as it was about helping others."

Research abounds with examples of how helping others reduces feelings of hopelessness after a personal crisis. Here are a few examples:

- People who volunteer after a natural disaster report feeling more optimistic and energized, and less anxious, angry, and overwhelmed, by the stress in their lives.
- After the death of a spouse, taking care of others reduces depression.
- Survivors of a natural disaster are less likely to develop posttraumatic stress disorder if they help others in the immediate aftermath.
- Among people living with chronic pain, becoming a peer counselor relieves pain, disability, and depression and increases sense of purpose.
- Victims of a terrorist attack feel less survivor guilt and find more meaning in life when they find a way to help others.

- After enduring a life-threatening health crisis, people who volunteer experience more hope, less depression, and a greater sense of purpose.

Helping others doesn't just transform the psychological impact of suffering; it also protects against the harmful effects of severe life stress on physical health. In fact, helping others seems to eliminate the impact of traumatic events on health and longevity.

In one groundbreaking study, researchers at the University at Buffalo tracked one thousand Americans between the ages of eighteen and eighty-nine for three years. Every year, the researchers asked the participants about stressful life events. They were interested in the big stressors that had happened that year—things like a family crisis, financial problems, or the death of a loved one. The researchers also asked how much time the participants spent giving back to their communities. Did they serve on the school board or a church committee? Did they do things to improve the neighborhood, like tend to a community garden or volunteer at a blood drive? Finally, they asked about participants' health. Had they been diagnosed with any new health problems? Not minor ailments like a cold, but serious problems like back pain, cardiovascular disease, cancer, and diabetes.

Among people who did not serve their communities in some way, every stressful life event, like a divorce or job loss, increased the risk of developing a new health problem. But there was no such risk for people who regularly spent time giving back. For them, there was zero association between stressful life events and health.

The same scientists conducted another study, this time looking at the effects of helping on longevity. The researchers tracked 846 men and women living in the Detroit area for five years. At the beginning of the study, the researchers asked participants how many major negative life events they had experienced in the past year. They also asked how much time the participants had spent helping friends, neighbors, and family members outside their immediate household. Then, over the next five years, researchers checked obituaries and official death records to find out who had died.

Once again, caring created resilience. Among those who did *not* routinely help others, every significant stressful life event increased the risk of dying by 30 percent. But participants who went out of their way to help others showed absolutely no stress-related increased risk of death. In fact, even when they had experienced several traumatic events, they had the same risk of dying as people who experienced no major stressful life events. They seemed to be completely protected from the harmful effects of stress.

Now, it's not the case that none of the caring folks died or developed any health problems. Helping others doesn't make you live forever, and it can't protect you from everything. But what it does protect you from is stress. In these two studies, the benefits of caring held for both men and women, among all races and ethnicities, and across the life span. Despite the widespread assumption that stress increases the risk of illness and death, this does not appear to be true for people who take a tend-and-befriend approach to life.

THIS CAN all sound very inspiring, especially if you already volunteer regularly and take great joy in giving back. But what if your instincts under stress aren't quite so altruistic? As we've seen, people do have different tendencies when it comes to how they respond to stress. If you are not a natural tend-and-befriender, will you still benefit from helping others?

The answer is a resounding yes. A study at the University at Buffalo directly addressed this question by collecting DNA samples from participants. The researchers looked at variations of a gene that influences how sensitive you are to oxytocin, the neurohormone that encourages a tend-and-befriend response. The researchers initially suspected that people who were more sensitive to oxytocin would benefit the most from giving back to their communities—but the opposite turned out to be true. Participants who were genetically biased *not* to have a tend-and-befriend response got the biggest health benefit of being prosocial.

The scientists speculated that caring for others can jump-start the oxytocin system, even if you have a genetic predisposition that makes a tend-and-befriend response less likely. This is consistent with the idea that what you do in life changes the nature of your default stress response. The act of helping others—whether through volunteering or simply connecting to your bigger-than-self goals—can unlock a biological potential for resilience.

"FROM THE COMMUNITY AND READY TO SERVE"

The link between caring and resilience suggests an intriguing possibility for how we can support those who have experienced severe stress or trauma. The best way to help these individuals, who are often labeled "at-risk," might be to turn them from victims into heroes, and to help them help others.

One program taking this approach is EMS Corps in Alameda County, California, which trains disadvantaged young men to become emergency medical technicians in their own communities. Many trainees live in high-poverty neighborhoods, where 60 percent of young men drop out of high school. Some trainees have been homeless. They are used to being viewed as a threat in their own communities; when they walk down the street or into a store, many people assume they are part of the gangs, crime, and violence that plague their neighborhoods. The lack of opportunities, compounded by the sense of being unwelcome in their own community, can easily push these young men toward a defeat response. Eventually, some of them become exactly the kind of problem to the community that others already see them as.

Alex Briscoe, the director of the Alameda County Health Care Services Agency, saw these young men differently. "The same young adults who have been vilified as noncontributing members to our society aren't actually the problem," he said. "They are the solution."

EMS Corps—whose slogan is "From the community and ready to serve"—is designed to change the way the community sees the young men, and how they see themselves. In addition to learning how to provide emergency care, the young men are put to work improving public health. For example, they provide free car-seat safety checks for parents and go door-to-door offering blood pressure readings and education on improving cardiovascular health. After one such event, when trainees lingered on a sidewalk in Berkeley, discussing the day's experiences, a young member of the EMS Corps said, "Giving them advice is a real good feeling."

The vocational training combined with mentoring is designed to help the young men develop an identity based on helping others. It's not just about teaching them how to respond to a person in crisis; it's also about using that role to develop courage, character, and commitment. As one trainee explained in a group mentoring session, "I learned the potential I have. I learned who I really am, and who I could become." A 2013 graduate of the program, reflecting on how the training affected his life, said, "I have the chance to be a real-life superhero." The graduates are also succeeding; 75 percent are employed in the field of emergency responding, and many are in college. That is an impressive outcome in an area where the unemployment rate for young men is as high as 70 percent.

RESEARCH SHOWS that this kind of intervention—helping the at-risk help others—can also reduce the negative health effects of poverty and chronic stress. In one study, students at an urban public high school in British Columbia, Canada, were randomly assigned to volunteer for one hour a week at an elementary school. Most of these teenagers were poor minority students with high levels of stress at home. Their volunteer time included helping elementary students with homework, sports, art, science, or cooking. After ten weeks, the teens who had volunteered showed improvements in cardiovascular health, including lower cholesterol and reduced levels of two markers of inflammation, interleukin-6 and C-reactive protein. The control group showed no changes.

The researchers also looked at whether any psychological changes could explain the biological ones. The students who reported the greatest increase in empathy and desire to help others showed the greatest reduction in cholesterol and inflammation. Volunteering also improved the teens' self-esteem, but greater increases in self-esteem were not associated with greater health improvement. The protective effect of volunteering came from a tend-and-befriend mindset.

Programs based on caregiving have even become first-line treatments for post-traumatic stress disorder. The Warrior Canine Connection in Brookeville, Maryland, for example, enlists soldiers with PTSD or traumatic brain injuries to train service dogs for other veterans. The soldiers bond with the dogs, while also serving the bigger mission of helping their fellow wounded warriors. The veterans who participate in the program report a decrease in depression, intrusive memories, and self-medication—and a greater sense of purpose and belonging.

Too often, those who are underprivileged or are survivors of chronic or traumatic stress are seen only as victims, damaged by their experiences and having little left to offer. Ironically, interventions that reinforce this view may do more harm than good if they make the recipients feel like second-class citizens in their communities. Interventions that recognize survivors' strengths, and put those resources to work, offer a promising counterbalance to the psychological toll of always being the one in need of help.

FROM PREDATORS TO PROTECTORS

> *I held his hand and said a prayer for him and said, "This pain and suffering is about to be over." I put his hat on him and covered him up with his blankets. He always liked sports, so I put the TV on ESPN. I kissed him on the forehead before I left.*

The man who described this moment of caregiving is not a relative of the patient, nor a nurse or hospice care provider. He is an inmate at a state correctional institution in Pennsylvania, caring for a fellow inmate who is dying. The story is one of dozens that have been told to Pennsylvania State University nursing researcher Susan Loeb, who studies end-of-life care in prisons.

Ask people where the tend-and-befriend instinct is least likely to be found, and a state penitentiary would surely make the list. Prison life requires a survival mentality. Many inmates grew up in harsh environments that rewarded self-defense over altruism. They may not have received consistent caregiving or had role models for compassion.

And yet compassion can flourish at prisons that provide inmates with caregiving opportunities, as Loeb has documented. She interviewed male inmates ranging in age from thirty-five to seventy-four who were providing care to dying prisoners at state correctional institutions. Most of these inmate caregivers are on call 24/7, with duties that range from making beds to changing adult diapers. They provide emotional support by talking, praying, holding hands, and helping the inmates prepare for visits from family. The caregivers also protect the dying inmates from predatory abuse by other inmates and act as intermediaries with correctional officers. The caregivers help keep the dying inmates comfortable at the end of their life, sit vigil, and help the medical staff provide after-death care.

Their reasons for getting involved are as noble as any you'll find outside prison: They want the opportunity to do something good, and they want make a difference. They understand that they themselves could be in the same boat as the dying inmates. One inmate caregiver was motivated by the memory of hearing a prison nurse issue these last words to a dying inmate: "Get ready to meet Satan." The inmates want to make sure that every prisoner is treated with dignity and kindness in his final moments.

Inmate caregivers are almost never paid for their work, nor do they receive special privileges. You might assume this would decrease their interest in participating, but it has the opposite effect. Without extra perks, the inmates can truly see themselves as compassionate caregivers. As one wrote in an anonymous survey, it was important to him "to give of my time without a need to be applauded or given certificates. To love others just because it's the right thing to do." When inmate hospice volunteers are asked, "What is the most important thing for people to know and understand about prison hospice and your volunteer work?" the most common response is the desire for people to know that they are helping because they really care. Many inmates say that caregiving allows them to express their true self. One told Loeb, "I was a predator. Now, I'm a protector." Another said, "I found something that I thought I'd lost in myself. I'm not a throwaway object. I got something to contribute."

Caregiving also transforms how the inmates experience their imprisonment. Even though they themselves are the ones providing compassion, the inmates witness fellow inmates receiving compassion. This shifts their perception of the prison system from one that is completely dehumanizing to one that does, at least in this one way, honor their humanity. Their own contributions end up changing how they experience the system they live in. In this respect, the inmates become recipients of their own caregiving.

As Susan Loeb told me, "People say, 'We could never do this here. It won't work,'" when they hear about inmate caregiving. I've heard that kind of assumption, too—not from prison management, but from people who assume that their coworkers, students, or other communities would have no interest in caring for others. And yet the benefits of connecting to the tend-and-befriend response are not limited to those places and people we traditionally associate with compassion. When given the opportunity, people in difficult circumstances often leap at the chance to help others.

If there's one thing we've seen in all these studies and stories, it's that the instinct to help is part of what it means to be human. Compassion is not a luxury reserved only for those with an easy life, nor is it just the province of saints and martyrs. Caring can create resilience and provide hope even in the most unexpected places.

When You Feel Alone in Your Suffering

Several years ago, I was walking home from the grocery store when I heard someone call my name. I turned around to see a Stanford graduate student from one of my classes waving and running toward me. I didn't know her well, since she typically kept to herself in the back of the classroom. I expected to exchange a simple "Hello! How are you?" and go on my way. But when the young woman reached me, she broke into tears. Startled, I gave her a hug and asked her if she was OK. "I'm just so lonely," she said. Then she told me something that broke my heart. "And you always seem so happy. I don't know how you do it."

This student knew me in only one context—teaching. In that role, my own suffering is less visible. But of course, just like her, I know what loneliness feels like. And when I was a student, there were days when I cried because I wanted to be happier but didn't know how. In fact, I remember my first Thanksgiving at Stanford—I had been so busy working that I hadn't made many friends in the three months I'd been on campus. On Thanksgiving Day itself, the campus was mostly deserted, so I went for a walk around town. I couldn't find anyplace that was open to grab a coffee or meal. When I finally walked back toward my campus apartment, it was dark out. As I passed by the student union, I saw a group of students sitting around a table in the middle of a Thanksgiving feast. I remember very clearly looking in that window and feeling like I was the only one who was alone and lonely on campus that day. I can look back now and realize that wasn't true, but sometimes, when you don't have a lot of support around you, it is easy to feel like you are the only one struggling.

The sense of being alone in our suffering is one of the biggest barriers to transforming stress. When we feel isolated and disconnected, it is more difficult to take action or see any good in our situation. It also can keep us from reaching out to others, either to get the help we need or to benefit from being of help to others. The ironic thing is, probably nothing is more universal than the experience of stress. Nobody gets through life without experiencing physical pain, illness, disappointment, anger, or loss. The specifics may vary, but the underlying experience is as human as it gets. The challenge is to remember this in your own times of suffering.

A MINDSET OF ISOLATION OR COMMON HUMANITY

Look at the four statements below and consider which pair feels more true for you:

- When I'm feeling down, I tend to feel like most other people are probably happier than I am.

- When I'm really struggling, I tend to feel like other people must be having an easier time of it.

- When I'm down, I remind myself that there are lots of other people in the world feeling like I am.
- When things are going badly for me, I see the difficulties as a part of life that everyone goes through.

These items are taken from a measure of what psychologists call *common humanity*—the degree to which you see your own struggles as part of the human condition. The first two items reflect a mindset of isolation, while the second two demonstrate the ability to feel connected to others even in your darkest moments. Importantly, these two mindsets have very different consequences. People who feel alone in their stress are more likely to become depressed and to rely on avoidant coping strategies, including denial, giving up on their goals, and trying to avoid stressful experiences. They are less likely to tell others about their stress and suffering, and so are less likely to receive the support they need. This makes them even more convinced that they are alone in their struggles.

In contrast, people who understand that suffering is part of everyone's life are happier, more resilient, and more satisfied with life. They are more open about their struggles and more likely to receive support from others. They are also more likely to find meaning in adversity and less likely to experience burnout at work. And yet, despite the benefits of recognizing common humanity, people often underestimate the stress in other people's lives and overestimate other people's happiness. This is true not just with strangers, but also with neighbors, coworkers, and even sometimes friends and family we think we know well. In *The Mindful Way Through Anxiety*, psychologists Susan Orsillo and Lizabeth Roemer describe this fundamental confusion:

We often judge our insides, which we know intimately, by other people's outsides, because that is all we can see. Often we are surprised and taken aback to find a coworker is struggling with suicidal thoughts, a neighbor has a drinking problem, or the lovely couple down the road engages in domestic violence. When you ride with people on the elevator or exchange pleasantries in the line at the grocery store, they may appear calm and in control. Outward appearances do not always reflect the struggles within.

Because the suffering of others can be less visible to our eyes, we often look out at the world and conclude that we are alone in suffering.

Research shows that modern forms of communication contribute to this misperception by encouraging us to present a positive picture of our lives. People prefer, or feel pressured, to post good news, happy photos, and positive milestones on social media. Even though most people are aware of their own tendency to do this, they underestimate the degree to which others are also putting on a positive show. So you can find yourself scrolling through upbeat posts from friends and family, wondering why your life is so much more chaotic, disappointing, or difficult than theirs. This misperception leads to a greater sense of isolation and less satisfaction with life. Studies show that spending time on social media, including Facebook, can increase loneliness and decrease satisfaction with life. The tendency to view our own lives as less happy than other people's lives is likely one reason why.

So how do you find a mindset of common humanity if what you usually feel is isolated by your problems? This is a question I've explored in my own research developing mindset interventions through Stanford's Center for Compassion and Altruism Research and Education. I've found that to feel less alone in your stress, two things help: The first is to increase your awareness of other people's suffering. The second is to be more open about yours.

Making the Invisible Visible

One of the exercises I use with groups to increase a mindset of common humanity is something I call "making the invisible visible." I ask everyone in the room to write on a slip of paper something they have struggled with and that continues to affect them now, *but that no one would know just looking at them.*

After everyone writes something down, I collect the slips and mix them up in a bag. We then stand in a circle and pass the bag around. Each person pulls an anonymous slip out of the bag and reads it out loud, as if it were his or her own. "I am in so much physical pain right now, it is hard for me to stay in this room." "My only daughter died ten years ago." "I worry that I don't belong here, and that if I speak up, everyone will realize that." "I am a recovering alcoholic, and I still want a drink every day."

Going through this exercise is profound on many levels. First, because the slips are anonymous, it is impossible to know whose statement is whose. And without fail, the statement that each person randomly draws seems as though it could truly be his or her own truth. Second, it makes visible so much of the suffering that was previously invisible. It was all already in the room, but because it was unspoken, it went unrecognized. In that invisibility, each person's individual suffering can feel isolating, but once it is named, it becomes a reminder of common humanity. Whenever I find myself feeling alone in any particular struggle, I try to recall the feeling of standing in one of these circles and the awe that arises when the previously unseen pain and strength of others is made visible.

You don't need to do this formal exercise in a group to benefit from the idea behind it. Whenever you are in a group, you can simply think about what is invisible. I recently heard a sermon by Pastor Karen Oliveto at Glide Memorial Church in San Francisco that gave this same advice. "Life isn't easy for any of us," she reminded the congregation. "If you think that if only you had the life of the person sitting down the pew from you—you know nothing of that person's life. Because, truth be told, that person possesses burdens you can't even believe. Each of us carries our private heartache, is tormented by our personal demons, is overwhelmed by the demands of our day when we simply cannot take on another thing or our backs will break."

One phrase I say to myself to remember this truth is, "Just like me, this person knows what suffering feels like." It doesn't matter who "this person" is. You could grab any person off the street, walk into any office or any home, and whoever you find, it would be true. Just like me, this person has had difficulties in his or her life. Just like me, this person has known pain. Just like me, this person wants to be of use in the world, but also knows what it is like to fail. You don't need to ask them if you are right. If they are human, you are right. All we need to do is choose to see it.

A Sleepless Night Before Surgery

One of my students, Cynthia, was in the hospital for a routine surgery. The night before the surgery, she couldn't sleep. Even though everyone expected the surgery to go well, it required general anesthesia. Cynthia was anxious about being put under, worrying about all the things she couldn't control. She was a mom, and worst-case scenarios always found their way into her thinking. Since she was awake, and the worrying wasn't helping, Cynthia decided to try thinking about common humanity.

First, she thought about the surgery itself and the anxiety she felt about not being able to control the experience. Then she brought to mind all the other people who were also facing medical procedures they might feel anxious about. People who had to start another round of chemo tomorrow. People waiting for the results of medical tests. People who didn't even know if they would be able to get treatment. People without insurance, waiting on a transplant list, or trying to get into a clinical trial. She thought about all that anxiety and about how many countless people were in the same boat with her. She felt a sense of connection to them. The awareness of even a nameless, faceless community who shared her same feelings was reassuring.

Then Cynthia thought about her present experience of not being able to sleep because of worry. She thought about how many other people were probably awake at that very moment, also kept up by fear or worst-case thinking. How many other people had to get up the next morning to do something they didn't want to do? Not just surgery, but anything. An exam. A difficult conversation. Burying a loved one. This experience of lying awake, as alone as she felt, connected her to countless other people who were sharing this experience with her. Cynthia was struck by how brave they all were, and felt a sense of her own bravery by extension. She chose the phrase "May we all know our own strength" as an offering to all of them, herself included. When she got out of bed the next morning, she had the feeling that she was one of many, part of a group of people choosing to face that day's challenges.

Transform Stress: Turn Isolation into Common Humanity

When you feel isolated or alone in your suffering, try connecting to the truth of common humanity.

First, allow yourself to feel whatever thoughts and emotions come up when you think about your own situation. Acknowledge whatever the underlying pain is: anxiety, physical pain, anger, disappointment, self-doubt, or sadness.

Then consider the possibility that this source of suffering is part of the human experience. Just like you, countless other people know what it's like to feel this pain, regret, sadness, injustice, anger, or fear. It can help to bring specific examples to mind—situations that aren't identical to yours but that involve the same kind of pain or stress. Allow yourself to feel a natural sense of empathy for these people—an understanding of what they must be feeling in their own situations.

I like to end this reflection with a phrase that captures the sense of shared experience. One of my favorites is "May we all know our own strength." Some phrases my students like include "May we all find peace," "May we all be supported through this suffering," and "May we all know that we are not alone." In this way, you bring in a bit of the hope and courage that feeling connected provides.

Create the Supportive Community You Want

Lennon Flowers was twenty-one when her mother died of lung cancer. The loss changed everything about her life, and yet, when she graduated from college and moved to California, she found it difficult to talk about it. Everyone who had known her mother was on the other side of the country. The moment Flowers mentioned that her mother had died, she got one of two responses. Many people found a reason to disappear. The rest put on the pity face. Lips pursed into a frown, eyebrows flattened, head tilted slightly, and then always the same three words: "I'm so sorry." Both responses felt isolating. Either she was a burden to others, making them uncomfortable, or an object of pity. So, she learned to keep her story to herself, even though it felt like she was holding back an important part of who she was.

One day, when she was twenty-five, Flowers was apartment hunting with Carla Fernandez, a woman she had worked with and been friends with for months. Somehow it came out that Fernandez had lost her father. It was a huge point of connection for the two women; and yet, Flowers and Fernandez were both so good at avoiding the topic that it had taken months for them to recognize their shared experience of loss.

This was an aha moment for both women, who had felt isolated in their grief but wary of sharing their stories. Fernandez decided to host a get-together for all the young women she knew who had lost a parent. Four invitations were extended and accepted. Fernandez prepared paella from a family recipe, to honor her father, who was Spanish. The women ate on Fernandez's deck and talked until two in the morning.

This was 2010, and it was the first of what would become known as the Dinner Party. Now, Dinner Parties take place across the United States, each hosted by someone who has lost a loved one, and open to anyone who wants a safe place to talk about life after loss. Flowers and Fernandez cofounded the Dinner Party as a grassroots organization to help people who felt isolated by loss build their own communities. Through their website, they play matchmaker between hosts and guests and provide hosts with guidelines for creating a safe and supportive environment for honest conversation.

Every dinner is run as a potluck for up to ten people, many of whom meet for the first time at the party. Each guest is encouraged to bring a dish that can start a conversation about the loved one they lost: your sister's favorite lasagna; the cake your wife baked for your anniversary every year; the soup your father used to make for you when you were sick. The host gently guides the conversation over dinner, leaving room for guests to reflect on anything they want to talk about. There is laughter, and tears, and silence. Every dinner ends with a reflection by each guest on what they appreciated about the conversation and the community.

More recently, the group has begun to host dinners that bring together people who have experienced loss with those who want to learn how to better support them. At these events, guests share stories about what people did that truly supported them after a loss. *People ask about my dad's life and not just his death. People kept calling, even though I didn't call back. People joined me in reminiscing about my husband and were not afraid to say his name. People did not fall out of my life.* These stories, captured at parties and now shared online, have become a resource for people who want to help but don't know how.

For Flowers, creating the Dinner Party has helped in unexpected ways. "Loss can feel very paralyzing," she told me. "People find value in being valuable to others. It's been profound for me to move from a place of feeling very adrift in the world to find that purpose reinstated though the Dinner Party."

PEOPLE WHO want to feel more connected, supported, and cared about often believe they need to wait for someone else to come and offer those things first. One of the most helpful mindset shifts you can make is to view yourself as the source of whatever support you want to experience. The Dinner Party is an example of what it means to be the starting point of a supportive community. Flowers and Fernandez felt isolated by loss. They wished it were easier to talk about loss, and they wanted other people to talk more openly about it with them. So they started the conversation and created those open communities for themselves and others.

Although it can be daunting to take that first step, choosing to be the starting point of what you want is the best way to create the supportive community you seek. Research shows that when you intentionally shift your focus toward supporting others, you end up the recipient of more support. When you make an effort to express your gratitude, you end up being more appreciated by others. When you go out of your way to make sure others know that they belong, you become an important and cherished member of the community.

One of my students, Ariel, told me how she had discovered a more supportive community by finding the courage to talk openly about her struggles. Twelve years earlier, her thirteen-year-old daughter had told Ariel that she was a boy. The announcement was like a bomb exploding her sense of reality. It took Ariel and her husband several months to even begin to make sense of what was happening. For a while, they tried to process it on their own. But once Ariel and her husband decided to support their daughter's transition to identifying fully as boy, they knew they had to educate themselves about transgender issues.

As Ariel became a part of the community of parents with transgender children, she started getting invited to speak on panels. Soon she found herself supporting other parents as well. This is a great example of turning a personal crisis into an opportunity to connect. But what struck me most was when Ariel told me about an unexpected outcome of her willingness to go public with her story. Soon, parents all over town started sharing their own family experiences that they had previously kept hidden, out of shame and a sense of isolation. "Folks opened up with all sorts of uncomfortable secrets and shared how they had coped," Ariel told me. "Courage is contagious, to be sure!" (Another happy postscript: Her son, Ariel now proudly brags, has gone on to study nursing.)

When you feel isolated in your stress or suffering, consider what it is you most long for. If there is something that you want to experience, or a community you wished were available to you, how can you be the starting point of creating it for others? People who allow themselves to have a courageous vulnerability—to look first for how to support others, and to use their own suffering as the point of connection—end up receiving more social support themselves. Like Flowers, who cofounded the Dinner Party, and my student Ariel, who gave others permission to confess their own difficulties, they end up being the recipients of what they intended to create for others:

feeling less alone in their struggles and at the center of a caring community.

A HAND ON YOUR BACK

I was standing on the side of Huron Avenue in Cambridge, Massachusetts, watching runners cross the finish line of a five-mile race. It was a sunny, windy April morning.

A pack of teenagers stood on the other side of the road, all wearing royal blue shirts that said "Sole Train." Whenever another blue-shirt-clad runner neared the finish line, they went wild with cheers. "Bring it in!" These teens had finished the race but were sticking around to support their fellow Sole Train runners. The fastest of them had crossed the finish line at 35:22. At 1:09:09, one of the last runners appeared, struggling to maintain a slow jog. She was flanked by two other runners in blue shirts, each with a hand on her back. I recognized the two runners as young men who had finished first among the Sole Train teens. They had run back to find team members who were struggling. They literally had her back. When she finally crossed the line, the sideline crowd cheered as if she had won the race.

Watching the runners, I was filled with joy, and found myself wishing I were part of the community, not just an observer for the day. Sole Train is a running and mentoring program for Boston youths, supported by the Trinity Boston Foundation. I was introduced to the group through Natalie Stavas, the doctor who saved lives after the Boston Marathon bombing. I didn't know much about the program when I visited the five-mile race, but it quickly became one of my favorite examples of how to create a tend-and-befriend culture to support resilience in the midst of great adversity.

Jess Leffler, the director of Sole Train, started the program in 2009 after working as a counselor and an art therapist with at-risk youths through Trinity Boston Foundation. She had the idea for Sole Train while running the Chicago marathon in 2007. The heat was so extreme that half the runners withdrew from the race. Cops were yelling at the marathon runners, "You must stop running!" But Leffler persevered. It was incredibly difficult, but also an amazing experience of her own capabilities. As she was running, she thought about the kids she had been working with. They lived in poor neighborhoods with limited opportunities. Leffler wondered what this experience—training for a marathon and doing something you never thought you could do—would be like for them.

A year and a half later, she invited some teens to train with her for a half marathon. What started as a whim has since turned into a full-fledged program, with about 150 youths (called *young soles*) recruited from local schools and community services and 40 adult mentors (*old soles*) who volunteer and train alongside them. The program's mission is "Deconstructing Impossible." Leffler saw how many things that the youths she worked with believed were impossible, from escaping violence to graduating from college. "You achieve something you never thought was possible, and it opens everything," she told me.

What stands out most about Sole Train is the approach it takes to *how* the kids accomplish the seemingly impossible. Everything revolves around community and mutual support. The goal of every runner is not just to finish the race but also to help every member of Sole Train cross the finish. (The day I showed up for the race, the teens even encouraged me to run, despite the fact that they had never met me and I wasn't dressed for it.) "If you want to be competitive with yourself, that's great, have goals," Leffler said. "But never against someone else." By removing competition as the main goal, the training process becomes a mindset intervention to strengthen bigger-than-self goals.

I got to see this mindset put into practice when, before the race, the Sole Train runners gathered in a circle inside the community center that was hosting the run. One of the teens led the group in some yoga. After the stretching, a young woman walked the inside of the circle giving everyone a high five. When it was time to head out to the road, they got closer together and slung their arms around one another. Leffler offered some important pre-race reminders. Then all the runners took a turn saying one thing they were bringing to the group and one thing they'd like from the group. "I'm bringing my determination for everyone," one runner said. "What I need is someone slow and steady to run alongside me." Another teen said she was bringing her loud and crazy cheering, and wanted someone with a sense of humor to help her keep going when she got tired. Another was bringing his speed, so he could be the guy you want to pass on the way to the finish line.

The young soles support one another and their adult mentors, the old soles. Many of these mentors have never run and are in worse shape than the teens. During training or a race, they need as much encouragement as the younger runners. One of the mentors, Nate Harris, said that the blurring of who is mentoring whom is an important part of Sole Train. "They feel like they have something to offer you." Big-time lawyers and doctors run side by side with the youths. On the road, in sneakers and shorts, they are all just humans struggling to put one foot in front of the other. Leffler said this part of the program—making the at-risk youths equal to community leaders—is the most therapeutic intervention she's ever seen.

The approach Sole Train takes—inspiring a sense of personal possibility by fostering a mindset of connection—is supported by research. Students who feel supported and part of something bigger than themselves are also more likely to expect that they can improve their abilities through hard work and help from others. In turn, this leads them to engage more with challenges, rather than give up. To many of its young members, Sole Train provides proof of their own potential. One teen keeps all her race bibs on her whiteboard in her bedroom, so they can inspire her every day when she wakes up.

After all the runners had finished the five-mile race, Leffler called everyone together for a closing circle. Again, the group stood with arms around one another, despite now being coated with five miles' worth of sweat. One at a time, the runners shared how they were feeling. "I'm in pain, but I'm loving how I'm feeling," said one teen. Another offered, "I feel happy I finished—happy *we* finished." An adult runner shared, "I feel so blessed to be part of such a great group of people." As the circle of appreciation proceeded, the comments continued to reflect a mindset of connection. The post-race huddle ended with praise from Leffler. "I hope you're seeing now what you are capable of," she told the team, "and what is possible when you have the support of such an amazing group."

What struck me most, in observing the entire morning, was the utter lack of cynicism in the teens. They appeared to embrace the community-building rituals wholeheartedly. I also couldn't help noticing how much these teens reminded me of my best undergraduate students at Stanford. They showed leadership, kindness, and self-discipline. They were confident in how they interacted with their adult mentors. I wanted to spend more time around them and get to know them as individuals.

What's stunning is that many of these Sole Train runners attend a school in Boston referred to as the place of "last hope," where 90 percent of the school's students meet the diagnosis for post-traumatic stress disorder. Before Sole Train, some of these kids struggled to show up to school sober. Now they meet early for a seven a.m. run. In an environment where their strengths are acknowledged and needed, they flourish.

Final Thoughts

One evening when I walked into my New Science of Stress course, I found a newspaper waiting for me on the lectern. A student had brought in an article titled "Stress: It's Contagious" that appeared in one of our local papers. The article claimed that stress is "as contagious as any airborne pathogen" and compared its toxicity with that of secondhand smoke. One expert discussed a study showing that people had a stress response when they passively observed another person suffering. "It was surprising how easily the stress was transmitted," he said. Another expert urged people not to be "stress carriers." I later found another article online describing the same research; it led with the headline "Is Second Hand Stress Killing You?"

I was fascinated by how these articles not only reinforced the "stress is toxic" mindset but also added a new layer of threat: You can catch toxic stress by being around other people who are stressed, and your own stress is harming everyone around you.

When I read part of the article to my students and asked them what the practical takeaway was, the first response was, "Isolate yourself." Then, "If you are stressed, keep it to yourself. Don't share your worries with others." The lessons continued, all with the same themes: Stay away from people who are suffering. Don't let yourself get infected by being around people who are stressed. Don't be a burden to others by sharing your stress with them.

Of all the stress-will-kill-you scare stories I've ever seen in the media, this one saddened me the most. Because if you follow the strategies my students took away from the story, you'll cut yourself off from two of the most important sources of resilience: knowing that you aren't alone in your suffering and being able to help others.

The social nature of stress is not something to fear. When you take a tend-and-befriend approach, even contagious stress can be strengthening. As we've seen, caring creates resilience, whether the altruism is a response to rescue us from our own suffering or simply a natural reaction to the pain of others. A sympathetic stress response to another person's suffering can spark empathy and motivate helping, which in turn enhance our own well-being. Furthermore, we shouldn't be afraid to let others see the truth of our own struggles—especially when we need their support. In many ways, our transparency is a gift, allowing others to feel less alone and offering them the opportunity to experience the benefits of tending and befriending.

grow | *how adversity makes you stronger*

TAKE A MOMENT to identify a time in your life that was a period of significant personal growth—a turning point that led to positive changes or a newly found purpose.

When you have a specific period of your life in mind, then consider this: Would you also describe this time as stressful?

When I ask this question in workshops, almost everyone raises their hands to agree that, yes, the time that led to personal growth was also quite stressful. This is the paradox of stress on full display: Even if we would prefer to have less stress in our lives, it's the difficult times that give rise to growth.

The idea that we grow through adversity is not new. It's embodied in the teachings of every major religion and many philosophies. It has even become a cliché to say, "Whatever doesn't kill you makes you stronger." The latest science supports this notion. For example, when people are asked how they are coping with the biggest sources of stress in their lives, 82 percent say they are drawing on strength developed from past stressful experiences. Even the most unwelcome experiences can lead to positive change. Adversity can create resilience, and trauma often inspires personal growth.

Importantly, research also shows that choosing to see this side of stress can help you learn and grow. To find the courage to grow from stress, you need to believe that something good can come from your suffering. You also need to be able to see and celebrate the positive changes in yourself as you grow from the experience. And yet, when you are actually going through a situation difficult enough to elicit the "Whatever doesn't kill you . . ." cliché from well-meaning strangers or loved ones, you may not be so inclined to see the upside of your situation.

The science, stories, and exercises in this chapter will help you cultivate a *growth mindset*—one that recognizes the natural human capacity to grow during times of stress. We'll explore how to discover this perspective even in the middle of circumstances where hope is hardest to find. Stories will play a special role in this process, as we consider how the stories you hear, and the stories you tell, can help you find meaning in suffering.

Throughout, we'll see one important theme over and over: The good that comes from difficult experiences isn't from the stressful or traumatic event itself; it comes from *you*—from the strengths that are awakened by adversity and from the natural human capacity to transform suffering into meaning. Part of embracing stress is to trust this capacity, even when the pain is fresh and the future uncertain.

Whatever Does Not Kill Us
Makes Us Stronger

Mark Seery, a psychologist at the University at Buffalo, keeps a framed print of a thirty-two-cent Iowa postage stamp featuring the 1931 painting *Young Corn* by Grant Wood in his office. Although

Seery has lived in Buffalo for a decade and made it his home, he keeps the painting in view because its rolling hills and cornfields remind him of where he comes from.

The importance of a person's past plays a central role in Seery's research. He is best known for a controversial paper published in 2010 titled "Whatever Does Not Kill Us," in which he challenged the widespread belief that traumatic events always increase the risk of depression, anxiety, and illness. Instead, he showed that a history of negative life events can actually protect against these outcomes. Adversity, he claimed, can create resilience.

These surprising findings came from a study that tracked more than two thousand Americans for four years. It was a nationally representative sample, meaning that the age, sex, race, ethnicity, socioeconomic status, and other demographic details of participants mirrored those of the entire United States. As part of the study, researchers asked participants if they had ever experienced thirty-seven different negative life events, such as a serious illness or injury, the death of a friend or loved one, a major financial difficulty, divorce, living in an unsafe home or neighborhood, being the victim of physical or sexual violence, and surviving a natural disaster like a fire or flood. Participants could report more than one of each type of event, allowing for a wide range of total past adversity. On average, participants reported eight such events. Eight percent of participants reported not experiencing any of these events, and the maximum number reported was seventy-one.

To test the long-term effects of adversity, Seery looked at whether the number of traumatic events people had lived through predicted their well-being over the four-year study. One possibility was a direct and negative relationship: the more adverse events, the lower a person's well-being. Instead, Seery found a U-shape curve, with those people in the middle the best off. People who had experienced a moderate level of adversity had the lowest risk of depression, the fewest physical health problems, and the greatest satisfaction with life. People at the extremes—either the lowest or highest levels of adversity—were more depressed, had more health problems, and were less satisfied with their lives. Although many people idealize a life without adversity, those who actually have one are less happy and healthy than those who have faced some hardship. In fact, people with no trauma in their past are significantly less satisfied with their lives than people who have experienced the average number of traumatic events.

In follow-up surveys over the years, participants were also asked how they were coping with more recent stress. Had they experienced any new serious adversities since the last survey? If so, how had those events influenced their well-being? The consequences of a new traumatic event depended on a person's past. Participants with a history of adversity were less likely to become depressed or develop new health problems than those with a limited experience of adversity.

For all these outcomes, the protective effect of adversity was true for men and women, all ages, and all ethnicities and races. Further, the effect could not be explained by differences in education, income, employment, marital status, or other social factors. Whatever the most difficult experience of a person's life, there was a good chance that it made that person stronger.

ARE YOU SAYING I SHOULD GIVE THANKS FOR MY SUFFERING?

Most of the feedback Seery has received on his findings has been positive, including many grateful emails from people who believe that the struggles in their past have made them stronger. They appreciate that Seery's research gives them a way to describe to others what they've witnessed in themselves.

However, Seery's work also has the potential to offend. When he first submitted the paper for publication in a scientific journal, one reviewer rejected the paper, claiming that Seery was endorsing child abuse. The reviewer told Seery, "You're saying these negative events are good, and that's dangerous." I've had similar experiences simply describing Seery's findings to others. At a conference for people who work with trauma survivors, a fellow speaker publicly criticized me for talking about Seery's work in my presentation on resilience. He thought I was implying that people who had been raped, abused, or otherwise victimized should be grateful for the opportunity it gave them to grow.

When I reported the pushback I had gotten, Seery sympathized but rejected the interpretation. "I just look at it so differently," Seery told me. These negative events are so unambiguously bad at the time they occur, he explained, that there is no denying that. It's easy to see the negative in suffering. "The tricky part," he added, "is to see anything other than that."

Seery isn't endorsing trauma. He simply wants to figure out the role that adversity plays in the human experience. He understands that most people would prefer to hand their traumatic experiences back to the universe. And he's certainly not suggesting we stop trying to prevent suffering so that people have more opportunity to develop resilience. But as much as we want to avoid pain and suffering, it's almost impossible to get through life without experiencing some trauma, loss, or serious adversity. If avoiding suffering isn't possible, what is the best way to think about the experience? "Given that it's happened," Seery asked, "does it mean your life is ruined?" He thinks his work gives a very clear answer. "People are not doomed to be damaged by adversity."

AFTER HIS controversial 2010 paper, Seery took his research into the laboratory. If adversity really makes people more resilient to future stress, he thought, he should be able to observe this resilience in action during stressful situations. How do people with a difficult past respond to pain or psychological pressure? And do their responses differ from those of people who have suffered less?

If you were a subject in one of Seery's studies of resilience, you might experience this: You come into the laboratory and are asked to sit in a plastic chair that reminds you of a doctor's office. On a table next to you is a large plastic container filled with water chilled to one degree Celsius (thirty-four degrees Fahrenheit). How cold is this? Consider the fact that human tissue begins to freeze at ten degrees Celsius. Below five degrees, water becomes so painfully cold that it feels like it is burning your skin. If you were to immerse your whole body in water this cold, it would kill you in less than a minute.

The experimenter asks you to dunk your hand in the water and place your palm on a large X on the bottom of the container. Already, your hand and arm are in pain. "We'd like you to hold your hand in the water as long as you can stand it," the experimenter says. "But you can choose when to stop. When you can no longer stand having your hand in, take it out. You don't need to ask permission, and there is no cost to stopping."

Once your hand is in the water, the experimenter asks you two questions every thirty seconds: On a scale of one to ten, how strong is the pain? On a scale of one to ten, how unpleasant is the pain? The test ends when you pull your hand out of the water, or when you reach five minutes (any longer could cause permanent damage).

In this study, Seery was interested in two aspects of resilience: How long can you withstand the pain, and how much does it upset you? Once again, he found evidence that adversity can make you resilient. Participants unfamiliar with adversity found the cold to be the most painful and unpleasant and took their hands out the fastest. People who had faced the most adversity kept their hands in the longest.

Seery also asked participants what they had been thinking during the pain. Those who had experienced the least adversity were more likely to think things like *I kept wishing that it would be over. I thought that the pain might overwhelm me. I felt that I couldn't stand it. I couldn't stop thinking about how much it hurt.* This kind of thinking—what psychologists call catastrophizing—not only makes a difficult experience more distressing, but it also makes you more likely to give up. In this study, catastrophic thinking explained the relationship between a person's past adversity and his or her ability to tolerate pain. Going through something difficult makes you less likely to catastrophize, and that gives you greater strength.

Although this experiment shows us just a thin slice of how participants respond to stress, these effects can add up in the real world. For example, among adults with chronic back pain, those with a history of moderate adversity report less physical impairment, rely less on prescription pain medication, have fewer doctor visits, and are less likely to be unemployed due to disability. They are handling the physical pain better and are less likely to have their lives disrupted by it. Police officers who have experienced at least one traumatic event before joining the police service show greater resilience following a traumatic event on the job, such as witnessing a fatal car accident or the death of a fellow officer. They report fewer symptoms of post-traumatic stress and are more likely to report positive outcomes from the trauma, such as an increased appreciation for life. When life has tested your strength, you are more likely to know that you can handle the next challenge, and your past experience can become a resource for coping.

Out of curiosity, I took the cumulative lifetime adversity measure to see where I fit in these research findings. I—like many of my students and the individuals I work with as a health psychologist—have experienced more negative events than is, per Seery's analyses, ideal. According to his findings, I might be happier or healthier if I had been spared some of those life events and losses. And yet, even though I don't land in his statistically ideal zone of resilience, I still find this research inspiring. There is a big difference between believing that every adversity has weakened me and knowing that some of these experiences have strengthened me. When I'm going through a particularly difficult time, I find it helpful to view my past experiences as resources to help me through the current crisis.

This is one takeaway from Seery's research. And yet, sometimes people look at his findings and focus on the very far-right end of the U-shape curve—where people have experienced the most traumatic events and also the most ongoing distress. Those with the highest levels of past adversity are more likely to be depressed or have health problems than those who have experienced less suffering. Some people who encounter Seery's work read this part of his graphs as indicating a kind of breaking point. As if once you've experienced a certain amount of adversity, you're a broken human being. I asked Seery about this interpretation of his data. Did he agree with it? Did he view his research as evidence for an important cutoff—some adversity is good for you, but once you cross a certain threshold, you're screwed?

His response surprised me. First, he rejected the cutoff interpretation and the idea that his findings prove there is some optimal number of negative life experiences. "I look at it more as evidence that something that was unqualifiedly negative at the time doesn't have to stay damaging. There is a message of hope in that, for anyone, no matter where they find themselves on the scale."

Seery also told me that his models can't even make predictions for people who have experienced the greatest adversity. These folks are literally off the charts in terms of the trauma they've experienced. Because they are so far from the statistical average, and there are so few of them in any given study, it's impossible to confidently estimate the effect of experiencing that much adversity. Anecdotally, though, he said that when you look at them individually, they are not necessarily doing the worst among his study participants. Some are doing exceptionally well. "There's a lot of room left, even if someone has experienced a lot of adversity, to rise above that and not be irreparably damaged," he explained. "I don't have a clear answer for whether it happens on average, but I feel confident that it is possible."

Cultivating a Growth Mindset

Thirteen first-generation college students sat on sofas and chairs pushed together in front of me. We were in the basement of a sporting goods store in San Francisco. It was the end of summer, and the students were about to head off to campuses around the United States to start their freshman year. All thirteen were part of an organization called ScholarMatch, which provides college counseling, scholarships, and mentorship to promising students in the San Francisco Bay Area.

I was there to give a college success workshop. Later in the day, they would get practical advice on everything from personal finance to interacting with professors. Other college students who had been where they were only one or two years ago would dispense practical wisdom. But first, I was kicking the day off with a growth mindset workshop.

I started by telling the ScholarMatch students about my favorite undergraduate at Stanford. Because for several years I co-taught the Introduction to Psychology course, a popular class with freshmen, I got to know hundreds of students in their first year at Stanford. Luis stands out over all others. It started when he flunked the first exam.

Whenever a student failed an exam in the course, I always sent an email encouraging him or her to come see me during office hours. I told them about resources we had available, including myself, TAs, and peer tutors. And yet many students didn't respond, all but guaranteeing they would barely pass the course. A lot of students wrote back with explanations or excuses, seeming not to realize that I was offering help, not scolding them.

Luis responded immediately, and in a panic. He had studied hard and had no idea why he had failed. He showed up to my office hours with his textbook and notes, wanting to review the exam questions to see what he missed. We went over his lecture notes and talked about how to listen more effectively in class and take better notes. We discussed strategies for studying from the textbook. This wasn't a one-time office-hours appearance. Luis kept showing up, once a week. Sometimes we talked about other things, including his other coursework, how he was fitting in at Stanford, and how he didn't want to disappoint his family at home.

Luis ended up with a B in the course, which is the only time in my career that I've seen a student who failed the first exam make such a dramatic recovery. More important, I told the ScholarMatch students, I was invested in him. When he needed a letter of recommendation to become a resident assistant in his dorm, I was thrilled to write it. When he needed a reference for a summer fellowship, I jumped at the chance to support him. I was officially a champion for Luis. And it happened not because he was a natural superstar who aced the course. It happened because he turned an adversity into an opportunity. He let an F be a catalyst to draw on the personal strengths that had gotten him into Stanford, and to develop the skills and relationships he needed to succeed here.

Put yourself in his place, I told the ScholarMatch students. Can you imagine that failing the first exam of your college career could turn out to be one of the best things that could happen to you?

I had chosen this story to start the workshop because it is at odds with how so many young people are taught to think about failure. They view it as something to avoid at all costs because it will reveal that they aren't smart or talented enough. This mindset can creep in whenever we are at a growth edge, pursuing any goal or change that is beyond our current abilities. Too often, we perceive setbacks as signals to stop—we think they mean something is wrong with us or with our goals. This can trigger a vicious cycle of self-doubt and giving up. In fact, when I came to give this workshop to the ScholarMatch students, the staff were still shaken up by one of their student's recent reactions to a minor setback.

The student had received a scholarship to attend a private university across the country. While traveling to attend summer orientation at the school, he missed his connecting flight. This one setback—which wasn't his fault, and wasn't insurmountable—seemed to him like a sign. He became convinced that the missed flight meant he should not go away to a four-year school. He called the Scholar-Match office from the airport, distraught. He wanted to give up his scholarship, stay in California, and attend community college. Once he was back home, ScholarMatch counselors talked him through his decision, and he decided to stick with the four-year school. But what would have happened if that extra encouragement hadn't been available?

So, during my time with the soon-to-be freshmen, I wanted to help them adopt a growth mindset—to view setbacks as inevitable, and understand that hitting an obstacle means it is time to draw on your resources. After I shared Luis's story with the students, I explained how setbacks and failures can be catalysts for growth. The question, I told them, isn't if you will ever have a setback or challenge at college, but what you will do when it happens. Experiences that most students dread—critical feedback on a paper, not doing well on an exam—are, in a strange way, moments to look forward to. They are your invitation to start building resources on campus, just like Luis did. When he asked for help and put in the extra effort, he invested in himself, and I invested in him. He ended up not just with a good grade but also with someone who genuinely cared about him and would go the extra mile to help him succeed.

Then I introduced a storytelling exercise. I asked the Scholar-Match students to think of a time when they had experienced a setback or challenge and persevered. Maybe they did poorly in a class but ended up getting through in a way they were proud of. Maybe it was a time they were treated unfairly but didn't let it discourage them. Or maybe they got into a fight with someone they cared about but were able to repair the relationship. Then I gave them an example from my own life, about how I had almost quit graduate school.

Near the end of my first year at Stanford, I was analyzing a data set that our laboratory had been collecting all year when a lab assistant asked me a question about an inconsistency in the file. When I checked the file we were analyzing against the original data, I realized that I had made a technical error, more than two months back, merging several sources of data. My error had destroyed the fidelity of the data file we had been analyzing, and all the findings we thought we had observed were not, in fact, accurate. They were the product of a corrupted data set.

I was horrified by my error and thought it proved that I wasn't cut out for a PhD. This wasn't a new fear; I had worried the whole year that I would show my limits. Unlike most students, who proudly wore Stanford T-shirts and sweatshirts to class and around campus, I didn't own a single item with a Stanford logo. Instead, I was already anticipating the shame I would feel if I failed and had to leave the university—and I didn't want to feel foolish for having bought a Stanford hoodie.

Telling my advisor about my mistake was one of the hardest things I'd ever done. I actually thought it would be easier to quit the program and disappear. (After all, one of my fellow first-year PhD students had gone home for winter break and never come back. He sent his advisor an email that said, "Sorry, psychology research isn't for me!") But instead of hiding or slinking away, I sat down and explained what had happened. To his great credit, my advisor didn't chastise me for my mistake. Instead, he told me a story about a similarly disastrous research mistake he had made early in his career. He helped me fix the file and get the project back on track. In fact, the entire lab came together to help me finish my first-year project, and I received more empathy than the judgment I had anticipated.

After I shared this story with the ScholarMatch students, I asked them to spend a few minutes writing about their own experiences with setbacks. What had happened, and why was it important to them? What was it in them that allowed them to persevere—what beliefs, attitudes, or strengths did they draw on? (In my case, I relied on my values of honesty and courage.) And finally, did they draw on any resources or support from others (as I had with my advisor and labmates)?

Once everyone was done writing, we broke into small groups, and each student took a turn sharing his or her story. As the session went on, I heard tales of persevering despite racial discrimination, academic failures, family hardships, and strained friendships.

After everyone had a turn, each small group reported back to the whole group on what themes had emerged. One group said that what stood out most was a sense of common humanity. Although each individual story was different, everyone in the group had experienced failure, disappointment, and setbacks. Another group observed that the willingness to ask for help was the most important thing that had allowed them to succeed. The third group realized that adversity actually increased their positive motivation and made them want to work harder.

A few months after the workshop, I received a letter from one of the ScholarMatch freshmen. She wrote that while college was challenging and even harder than she had expected, she was persisting because she had learned that it was OK to ask for help.

THE KIND of workshop I led for ScholarMatch has been shown to help students respond more effectively to academic challenges. For example, after similar interventions at public schools in New York City and nearby suburbs (led by David Yeager and collaborators at Columbia University), students became more likely to revise assignments to improve their grades and to take a teacher's feedback. Because of this, their grades improved.

A growth mindset can also create resilience more broadly, especially among those who have faced early adversity. Edith Chen, a psychologist at Northwestern University, has identified a coping style called shift-and-persist that seems to protect people from the typical health risks associated with having grown up in poor or unsafe environments. *Shifting* is a combination of accepting stress and changing the way you think about its source. It's often measured by asking people how much they agree with statements like "I think about the things I can learn from a situation, or about something good that can come from it." *Persisting* is about maintaining the optimism needed to pursue meaning, even in the face of adversity. It is measured with statements like "I think that things will get better in the future" and "I feel my life has a sense of purpose."

People who cope with adversity by shifting and persisting seem immune to the toxicity of a difficult or disadvantaged childhood. Chen has studied children, adolescents, young adults, middle-aged adults, and older adults throughout the United States who grew up in what psychologists call risky environments. In every age group, those who report a shift-and-persist approach to stress are healthier. Chen uses a range of biological measures that are considered to reflect a toxic buildup of stress in the body, like blood pressure, cholesterol levels, obesity, and inflammation. Although a difficult childhood sometimes predicts unhealthier levels of all these factors, that is not the case for people who choose to see the meaning in stress and believe in their ability to learn and grow from it. They look as healthy as, or healthier than, people who had much less difficult childhoods.

Many things can affect whether someone uses a shift-and-persist strategy to cope with stress, including whether a child grew up with adults who modeled a growth mindset. But it's also something that can be cultivated at any stage of life, by choosing to appreciate how you have grown from adversity.

Transform Stress: Turn Adversity into a Resource

Bring to mind a stressful experience from your past in which you persevered or learned something important. Take a few moments to think about what that experience taught you about your strengths and how to cope with stress. Then, set a timer for fifteen minutes and write about the experience, addressing any or all of the following questions:

- What did you do that helped you get through it? What personal resources did you draw on, and what strengths did you use? Did you seek out information, advice, or any other kind of support?
- What did this experience teach you about how to deal with adversity?
- How did this experience make you stronger?

Now think about a current situation you are struggling through.

- Which of these strengths and resources can you draw on in this situation?
- Are there any coping skills or strengths you want to develop? If so, how could you begin to do so using this situation as an opportunity to grow?

Post-Traumatic Growth

During a recent New Science of Stress course, one of my students, Cassandra Nelson, told me about a particularly searing experience she and her husband had suffered through. She agreed to let me print their story in full, in her own words:

> During the forty-first week of pregnancy with my second child, I noticed that the baby's movement had stopped. Shortly after we arrived at the maternity ward at the hospital, my husband and I were told that our baby girl no longer had a heartbeat. Within twenty-four hours, the decisions to be made changed from what brand of diapers to use to whether we wanted an autopsy performed, and would we be cremating her body. We made it through a C-section delivery, where our beautiful, eight-and-a-half-pound baby girl emerged into the world, still and lifeless. She was wrapped in the usual baby print blanket and placed into our arms. We named her Margaux.
>
> Margaux had red hair and chubby cheeks, just like her big sister. She looked so peaceful, as though she was just sleeping. The flood of emotions was confusing and overwhelming. We cooed over her little features. My husband kept blurting out, "She's still amazing," as the nurse pushed him and Marguax out the door in a wheelchair, to wait for me to finish being stitched up.
>
> Once we got home, we toggled back and forth between being in a catatonic state and being angry, sobbing messes. We pushed ourselves to attend a grief support group offered by a local nonprofit organization, HAND of the Peninsula (Helping After Neonatal Death). Listening to the experiences of other couples, we discovered ways to keep the memory of our

daughter alive while simultaneously moving forward. Connecting with people through HAND helped us calm the fears about our future and created a sense of hope. We felt charged with the energy we needed as our lives shifted in new, unexpected directions.

My husband and I experienced huge changes in our lives following our loss. Toxic friendships began to dissolve. Longtime healthy friendships grew stronger, and amazing new friendships were born. Our personal values became more clear. I learned to forgive my body for failing to sustain the life of our child. I learned to love it again through yoga and painting. My husband began caring for his body through nutrition and exercise. Now over the age of forty, he is fitter than he has been since his twenties. At work, I accepted a more challenging position, something I would not have considered before our loss. I also began to care for my soul. I started studying and then converted to Judaism.

We found the courage to move forward with having another baby despite the fears and fertility issues that kept rearing their ugly heads. We finally got pregnant, stayed pregnant, and had our third child, a healthy boy.

My husband and I both discovered that our empathy had expanded. After our son was born, we began facilitating grief meetings for other parents who had lost a baby before or after birth. We wanted to help others who were struggling through the pain, as we had. We also began to feel more empathy for each other. Our relationship deepened. We put more energy into communicating with each other. We started to let go of the little things that used to make us feel fearful, angry, or irritated. More so now than ever, we feel deep gratitude and joy for the blessings in our lives, and truly enjoy the time that we get to spend with each other.

Many times I have reflected on how much I have grown through the experience of losing our daughter. At times, I feel guilty about how much my life has prospered following her death. This is usually followed by small affirmations from the universe that suggest my daughter's spirit is with me, always, cheering me on as I go. This feeling propels me further into being more engaged with life, and allows me to embrace life's challenges. The act of engaging makes me feel like my energy honors the memory of my daughter. Although her life was lost before she was born, it lit a fire within me that continues to illuminate.

Today, Nelson is a forty-two-year-old mother of three and a forensic scientist, and she continues to volunteer for HAND of the Peninsula in San Mateo, California. Nelson's story, while unique, reflects the stories of many people who have experienced a trauma or loss. The experience creates tremendous suffering, but at the same time, inspires positive change.

Psychologists call this phenomenon *post-traumatic growth*. Post-traumatic growth has been reported by survivors of almost every imaginable kind of physical and psychological trauma, including violence, abuse, accidents, natural disasters, terrorist attacks, life-threatening illness, and even long-term space flights. It has been documented among those who live with ongoing stress, such as caring for a child with a developmental disorder, adapting to a spinal cord injury, working as a trauma responder, and living with a chronic illness. And it is even reported by those who have experienced the most horrific traumas, including victims of rape and prisoners of war. Post-traumatic growth has been documented in children and adults, and in many cultures and countries, including the United States, Canada, Australia, the U.K., Norway, Germany, France, Italy, Spain, Turkey, Russia,

India, Israel, Iraq, China, Japan, Malaysia, Thailand, Taiwan, Chile, Peru, Venezuela, and more.

When people describe how they have grown from a traumatic event, they report the same kind of changes that Nelson and her husband experienced. Here are some of the most commonly reported forms of growth:

- I have a greater sense of closeness with, and compassion for, others.
- I discovered that I'm stronger than I thought I was.
- I have a greater appreciation for the value of my own life.
- I have a stronger religious faith.
- I established a new path for my life.

The prevalence of post-traumatic growth is hard to estimate. However, it is far from unusual: 74 percent of Israeli youths exposed to terrorist attacks report post-traumatic growth; 83 percent of women with HIV/AIDS report growth related to their diagnosis and illness; 99 percent of emergency ambulance workers report growth as a result of the trauma they are exposed to during work. As one 2013 review of research on post-traumatic growth declared, "Growth is not a rare phenomenon reported only by exceptional people."

POST-TRAUMATIC GROWTH doesn't mean that people bounce back from adversity, untouched by the trauma. Just because people are able to see positive changes in themselves or their lives doesn't mean they aren't still in pain. In fact, people routinely report both growth and harm from the same traumatic event. A 2014 analysis of forty-two studies even found that the severity of post-traumatic distress positively predicts the degree of post-traumatic growth. This has led many researchers to believe that post-traumatic distress and post-traumatic growth are not separate and unrelated phenomena. Instead, they argue that post-traumatic distress is the engine of post-traumatic growth. It ignites a psychological process that gives rise to positive changes.

That was the case for Jennifer White, who was twenty-three when her mother, Joanie, died by suicide in July 2011. Two years after her mother's death, she felt stuck in her grief. She had scattered her mom's ashes in a pond in Texas, gone to therapy, joined a support group, and participated in walks to raise awareness about suicide. But she was still angry and hurt, tired of wondering if she could have prevented her mother's death, and desperate to reconnect with her mother, somehow.

Then one day, White saw a call for volunteers to help paint an elementary school in Los Angeles, where she was living at the time. The announcement reminded her of the story of how her parents had first met at John Sealy Hospital in Galveston, Texas. Her mother was a nurse, and her father was completing his surgical residency, and the two met the day her mother volunteered to paint *Sesame Street* characters on the walls of the pediatric ward. To feel closer to her mother, White signed up to help repaint the elementary school. When she arrived, she was given one of the least glamorous jobs, scraping the old paint off an industrial grate that took up half the side of the building. White spent hours taking off paint with a tiny scraper as others went off to lunch. When it was done, she helped to repaint the grate bright blue.

In those hours, White felt more connected to her mother than she had in any moment since her mom's death. "I felt her there," White said. "It was something we would have done together." It was the first time since her mother's death that she had felt hope that she would be able to continue having a relationship with her mother, even after her death.

That day was a turning point for White. Soon after, she founded Hope After Project, a small organization that helps people plan service projects to celebrate the lives of their loved ones. She's organized a community garden project in East Harlem, a day trip to groom and feed kittens at Kitten Rescue in Los Angeles, a project to build and send care packages to men and women serving in the military, and a day of cleaning and cooking for cancer patients living at the American Cancer Society's Hope Lodge in Kansas City. White helps raise the funds to pay for the service projects, and friends and family of the person being celebrated are invited to participate. White describes her current life running Hope After Project as a complete 180-degree turn from the life she had been living before, as an actress in Los Angeles.

Despite appreciating these changes and the new meaning she had found in life, White was quick to point out that it doesn't undo the pain of her mother's death. "I like who I am better today than before she died, but that doesn't mean that I don't wish she were still here," White said. She was also very careful to point out, "It's not that my mom's death was good. I've found some good in it."

This is a critical distinction, and one of the most important things to understand about how adversity can make you stronger. The science of post-traumatic growth doesn't say that there is anything inherently good about suffering. Nor does it say that every traumatic event leads to growth. When any good comes from suffering, the source of that growth resides in *you*—your strengths, your values, and how you choose to respond to adversity. It does not belong to the trauma.

Choosing to See the Upside of Adversity

So far, we've seen that adversity can make you more resilient and that trauma can lead to growth. Moreover, we've seen that taking this point of view on your past challenges can help you persist in the face of present stress. But what about when you're in the middle of a stressful situation? Is there any benefit to believing that adversity helps you grow while you are neck-deep in it?

One way to answer this is to find people in stressful circumstances and ask them if they see any benefit in the situation. If they do, does it lead to a better outcome? The answer appears to be yes. Men who find an upside to their first heart attack—a change in their priorities, a greater appreciation for life, a better relationship with their family— are less likely to have another heart attack and more likely to be alive eight years later. HIV-positive women who recognize a positive outcome of their diagnosis—such as deciding to take better care of their health or to quit using drugs—have better immune function and are less likely to die of AIDS over a five-year follow-up. Among men and women with chronic pain or illness, seeing something positive in their suffering predicts improvements in physical function over time. In all these studies, researchers carefully controlled for participants' health status at the beginning of the study; seeing the upside in their health challenges was *not* a consequence of being healthier in the first place. Instead, seeing the upside first seemed to lead to these positive outcomes.

Finding the good in stress doesn't improve just physical health. It can also protect against depression and strengthen relationships. For instance, those who find a benefit in taking care of a spouse with Parkinson's disease—such as saying that they now have greater patience and acceptance or that they feel a stronger sense of purpose—are happier with their marriages, and so are their spouses. In teens with diabetes, benefit-finding reduces the risk of depression and also makes them more likely to comply with blood sugar monitoring and dietary restrictions. U.S. Army soldiers who see benefits in their deployment, agreeing with statements such as "This deployment has made me more confident in my abilities" or "I was able to demonstrate my courage," are less likely to develop post-traumatic stress disorder or depression. The protective effect is strongest for soldiers exposed to the most combat and trauma.

Why does seeing a benefit in these circumstances help? The biggest reason is that seeing the upside of adversity changes the way people cope. It's a classic mindset effect. People who find benefit in their difficulties report more purpose in life, hope for the future, and confidence in their ability to cope with the current stress in their lives. They then are more likely to take proactive steps to deal with the stress and to make better use of social support. They also are less likely to rely on avoidance strategies to escape their stress. Even their biological response to stress is different. In the laboratory, people who can find a benefit in their struggles show a healthier physical response to stress and a faster recovery. All this—rather than some sort of magical thinking—is why benefit-finding predicts outcomes as far-ranging as less depression, higher marital satisfaction, fewer heart attacks, and stronger immune function.

I have to admit that even as I write about this research, I struggle with the term *benefit-finding*. It bothers me in the same way that I've witnessed others object to *post-traumatic growth*, or to the cliché "Whatever doesn't kill you makes you stronger." To my ears, *benefit-finding* sounds like the kind of positive thinking that tries to scurry away from the reality of suffering: Let's look for the bright side so we don't have to feel the pain or think about the loss.

But despite my own allergic reaction, this research doesn't suggest that the most helpful mindset is a Pollyannish insistence on turning everything bad into something good. Rather, it's the ability to notice the good as you cope with things that are difficult. In fact, being able to see *both* the good and the bad is associated with better long-term outcomes than focusing purely on the upside. For example, people who report both negative and positive changes after a terrorist attack are more likely to sustain post-traumatic growth than those who initially report only positive changes, such as not taking life for granted anymore. The same is true for medical scares. Survivors of a life-threatening disease, as well as their caregivers, are more likely to experience lasting personal and relationship growth if they report both benefits, such as learning to live in the present moment, and costs, such as fatigue or fears about the future. Looking for the good in stress helps most when you are also able to realistically acknowledge whatever suffering is also present.

INVITING OTHER people to see the good in difficult circumstances is a tricky task, but some scientists have begun to show that it can transform people's experience of both ordinary, everyday stress and more severe suffering. In one study, researchers at the University of Miami asked people to think about a time when another person had hurt them in some way. The participants came up with juicy—and still painful—tales of infidelity, rejection, dishonesty, criticism, and disappointment. Then the researchers asked the participants to write for twenty minutes about how their lives were better as a result of the experience, or how the experience had helped them become a better person. After writing from this point of view, the participants were less upset about the experience. They felt more forgiving and less desire for revenge. They also reported less desire to avoid the person or any reminders of the experience.

Amazingly, another study found that even a two-minute version of this mindset intervention can transform the experience of thinking about a hurtful experience. In this study, conducted at Hope College (I know, perfect) in Holland, Michigan, participants were asked to do the following exercise:

For the next two minutes, try to think of [the experience] as an opportunity to grow, learn, or become stronger. Think of benefits you may have gained from your experience, such as self-understanding, insight, or improvement in a relationship. Actively focus on the thoughts, feelings, and physical responses you have as you think about ways you benefited from your experience.

During this two-minute reflection, participants were hooked up to an electromyography machine that measured the activity of individual facial muscles. Compared with participants who were asked to think about the hurtful experience without finding an upside, participants who thought about the benefits showed less tension in their brows and had greater activation of the zygomaticus major, the muscle in your cheek that lifts your mouth into a smile. In other words, their faces were happy. Even their cardiovascular responses were different. Without finding an upside, thinking about the experience resulted in a typical threat response—elevated heart rate and blood pressure. When participants contemplated the benefits, however, their hearts showed a tend-and-befriend response, one consistent with the physiology of gratitude and connection.

The mindset reset also transformed their mood. After the two-minute reflection, participants reported feeling less anger and greater joy, gratitude, and forgiveness. Importantly, they also felt a greater sense of control, which is likely one of the main ways benefit-finding leads to better coping. Separate studies show how this change plays out in the brain. Benefit-finding is associated with greater activity in the left frontal cortex, a part of the brain that has a major role in positive motivation and active coping.

Other mindset interventions take a long-term approach, like asking people to write or reflect on the benefits of a difficult situation every day for several weeks. After one such intervention on adults with autoimmune disorders such as lupus and rheumatoid arthritis, the participants reported reduced fatigue and pain. Those who struggled the most with anxiety before the intervention showed the biggest improvements in physical well-being. Women who wrote about the benefits of their cancer experience ended up reporting less distress and had fewer subsequent medical appointments for cancer-related problems. Tellingly, women who had been relying primarily on avoidance coping strategies, like denial and distraction, had the biggest reduction in distress.

Another intervention asked those caring for a relative with Alzheimer's disease to keep an audio diary of any positive caregiving experiences. Each night, they were to take a minute to record themselves talking about at least one uplifting caregiving experience of the day. At the beginning of the study, all the caregivers were mildly to moderately depressed. After several weeks of recording their audio diaries, they were significantly less depressed. The practice of seeing the daily uplifts in caregiving was more effective at reducing depression than a comparison intervention that focused on stress management.

In all these studies, the participants were confused at first. They had trouble even understanding the instructions. *You want me to write about the* benefits *of having cancer? The good parts of taking care of a husband with Alzheimer's disease?* They struggled to come up with anything to write or talk about. And yet, in each of these interventions, the participants came to appreciate the process. The ones who benefited the most were those who had been stuck in anxiety, avoidance, and depression. Seeing the upside doesn't fix a difficult situation, but it does help balance the distress with hope.

Despite the evidence that benefit-finding can help people cope, this is not a strategy to casually recommend to others. As one student memorably told me, if anyone ever suggested that she should find a benefit in the death of her husband, she would tell them to go to hell. I can appreciate this. Even therapists trained in benefit-finding are encouraged to simply listen for any benefits a client mentions and not to try to convince a client to see the upside of their suffering.

Transform Stress: Choose to Find an Upside in Adversity

Choose an ongoing difficult situation in your life or a recent stressful experience. What, if any, benefits have you experienced from this stress? In what ways is your life better because of it? Have you changed in any positive ways as a result of trying to cope with this experience?

Below is a list of the most commonly reported positive changes experienced in response to hardship, loss, or trauma. Consider whether you see any signs of these benefits in yourself:

- *A sense of personal strength.* How has this experience revealed your strength? Has this changed how you think about yourself and what you are capable of? How have you personally grown or changed as a result of having to cope with this experience? What strengths have you used to help yourself cope?

- *Increased appreciation for life.* Do you feel a greater appreciation for life or a greater enjoyment of everyday experiences? Are you more likely to savor simple moments? Do you feel more willing to take meaningful risks? Have you begun to give more time and energy to the things that bring you joy or matter most to you?

- *Spiritual growth.* In what ways has this experience helped you grow spiritually? Have you experienced a renewal of faith or reconnected with communities that are meaningful to you? Have you deepened your understanding of, or willingness to rely on, a religious or spiritual tradition? Do you feel that you have grown in wisdom or perspective?

- *Enhanced social connections and relationships with others.* How has this experience strengthened your relationships with any friends, family, or other members of your community? Has it given you more empathy for other people's struggles? Has it motivated you to make any positive changes in your relationships?

- *Identifying new possibilities and life directions.* What positive changes have you made in your life as a result of this experience? Have you set any new goals? Have you taken time to do things you might not have considered before? Have you found a new sense of purpose or been able to channel your experience into helping others?

That said, when chosen freely, benefit-finding can be very empowering. If you would like to try it, the mindset exercise on page 207 is a good place to start. Think of it as an exercise in being able to hold opposite perspectives at once, rather than an exercise in purely positive thinking. You don't need to talk yourself out of any distress you feel, or disregard any negative outcomes you've experienced. You're simply choosing to put your focus, for a brief period of time, on the good you see in the situation or in yourself as you cope with it.

I'm often asked if it is possible to find a benefit in *every* stressful experience—for example, is there an upside to being stuck in traffic? Maybe, but benefit-finding shouldn't be a knee-jerk response to every minor frustration. Trivial events are not great places to look for growth and positive change. If you try to find the benefit in them, it will be difficult to find an authentic answer. Not every trauma has an upside, either—and you shouldn't force a positive interpretation on every instance of suffering. Benefit-finding has the most power when a stressful experience has affected you deeply. It can also be especially helpful in situations you can't control, change, or leave. Although these may be the experiences you feel least able, initially, to see the benefit in, they are exactly the experiences that are most likely to be transformed by a willingness to look for growth and positive change.

When you first begin to look for the benefits in a stressful experience, you might find it challenging. As with any mindset change, it is natural to struggle with a new way of thinking. This exercise may be especially difficult if it feels like a denial of the harm or suffering you have experienced. If it feels that way to you, consider spending a few minutes writing about whatever thoughts and feelings come up, including any pain or distress, when you think about the experience. Then, if you feel willing, spend a few minutes writing about what growth or positive changes you would *like* to experience. At some point in the future, what change and growth might be possible?

How to Make Growth and Resilience Contagious

In 2002, Mary Wiltenburg, a twenty-six-year-old reporter for the *Christian Science Monitor*, spent a week with Sue Mladenik, a mother of four heading to Beijing to adopt a one-year-old girl. Mladenik was also a widow. Her husband, Jeff Mladenik, had boarded American Airlines Flight 11 from Boston to Los Angeles on the morning of September 11, 2001. Wiltenburg visited Mladenik's family for a story on the anniversary of the terrorist attacks—an update on how one person was coping one year later. As Wiltenburg recalled, Mladenik's pain was still right at the surface of every moment. She slept only a few hours most nights. Waves of grief flooded her in unexpected ways, like seeing Jeff's favorite cookie at the grocery store. She no longer took her youngest daughter to places like the zoo, where they would run into too many "mommy-daddy happy families." And she was angry at, not comforted by, the outpouring of well-wishers who made comments like "At least he's in a better place now."

The article Wiltenburg wrote about Mladenik's first year after

9/11 begins: "It took her five days to leave her bedroom, ten months to wash the sheets they'd slept in together, and more than a year to empty the dirty socks from Jeff's gym bag." It was an honest story about a family devastated by loss. The only thing keeping Sue alive was her responsibility to her five children, including the young girl she and Jeff had planned to adopt together.

After she filed the story, Wiltenburg was haunted by the overwhelming rawness of the suffering that was still very much present in the Mladenik family. For a long time afterward, the journalist had nightmares about plane crashes.

In 2011, Wiltenburg's editor asked if she would be willing to revisit the Mladenik family. How were they coping ten years after 9/11? Wilternburg jumped at the chance. This time, she met a family who continued to mourn, but who had also moved forward. Sue had adopted two girls from China and become a grandmother. In 2002, Sue had been dreading the first anniversary of the terrorist attacks. By 2011, the day had become a family holiday. Every September 11, "Team Mladenik" gets together to celebrate Jeff's life. For the ten-year anniversary, fifteen Mladeniks were planning to visit the 9/11 Memorial Museum and run a five-kilometer race in New York City in Jeff's honor.

Sue Mladenik told Wiltenburg she was less angry than she had been in 2002. She had rebuilt her life around her family, with the goal of making sure her children would remember their father. Sue had also found a new sense of purpose in life, dedicating her time to causes that she and Jeff had both supported. The pain was still there, and there were many moments of grief and confusion, but there was also meaning and a strong desire to face the future.

For Wiltenburg, this update to the Mladeniks' life was an important postscript to the original story of raw grief and senseless tragedy. Writing that story affected her as much as writing the 2002 article had, but this time, she was filled with hope instead of haunted by nightmares. "I feel that anyone, maybe even especially someone like me, whose losses have been smaller and less public, can learn from their story," Wiltenburg told me. "We are all broken people, in some way. For most of us, the big question is, how do you live a good life despite, or within, that brokenness? All of us are trying to figure out how to live with things that hurt."

IMAGES AND VOICES OF HOPE

Wiltenburg's ten-year follow-up of the Mladenik family is an example of a new type of journalism: restorative narratives. Restorative narratives reject the usual approach to reporting traumas and tragedies. Instead of sharing only the most horrific details of the immediate aftermath, they tell stories of growth and healing.

The reports we are exposed to in the media have a real impact on our well-being. In one major U.S. survey, exposure to the news was one of the most commonly reported source of daily stress. Of people who reported high levels of stress, 40 percent mentioned watching, reading, or listening to the news as a major contributor to the stress in their lives.

Stress caused by the news, as opposed to stress caused by your life, is unique in its ability to trigger a sense of hopelessness. Watching TV news after a natural disaster or terrorist attack has consistently been shown to increase the risk of developing depression or post-traumatic stress disorder. One shocking study found that people who watched six or more hours of news about the 2013 Boston Marathon bombing were more likely to develop post-traumatic stress symptoms than people who were actually at the bombing and personally affected by it. It's not just traditional news programs that instill fear and hopelessness; stories of tragedy, trauma, and threats dominate many forms of media. In fact, a 2014 study of U.S. adults found that the single best predictor of people's fear and anxiety was how much time they spent watching TV talk shows.

Findings like this motivate Images and Voices of Hope (IVOH), an organization dedicated to changing the way trauma, tragedy, and disaster are portrayed in the news. IVOH trains media professionals to tell stories of resilience and recovery. The organization has worked with journalists and photographers from major newspapers around the United States. The kind of restorative narratives that IVOH champions aren't fluff pieces that pretend that a person's or a community's suffering is over. However, these stories do choose to focus on the process of recovery. How do communities rebuild after a disaster? How do people re-engage with their lives after tragedy? How is meaning being created out of suffering?

According to Mallary Jean Tenore, managing director of IVOH, when people hear, read, or see restorative narratives, they feel more hopeful, courageous, and inspired to create change in their own lives. The resilience in the story is contagious. This is one of the great lessons of restorative journalism: There is power in the stories we tell and in the stories we pay attention to.

The idea that we can experience post-traumatic growth from other people's stories is not wishful thinking. New research shows that people can find meaning in, and experience personal growth from, the traumatic experiences of others. Psychologists call this "vicarious resilience" and "vicarious growth." It was first observed in psychotherapists and other mental health care providers, who often reported being inspired by their clients' resilience and recovery. Vicarious growth was most commonly reported by professionals working with people who had suffered greatly: nurses caring for severely injured children at a burn treatment center, social workers helping refugees and victims of political violence or torture, psychologists counseling bereaved parents. They spoke of finding hope and feeling better about their own capacity for resilience, as well as coping better with the challenges in their own lives.

Vicarious growth is not limited to those in the helping professions. One study, conducted by researchers at Bond University in Australia, asked adults to describe the most traumatic event they had been vicariously exposed to in the past two years. Participants reported events such as a miscarriage, surviving an accident, the death of a loved one, a serious illness, or crime. The events happened to friends, family members, spouses, or even strangers—some were learned about through the news. The participants reported not only vicarious growth, but also that this growth enhanced their ability to find meaning in their own lives.

How do you catch resilience and growth from another person's suffering, instead of only sympathetic distress? The most important factor seems to be a genuine empathy. You must be willing to feel their distress and imagine yourself in their experience. You also must be able to see their strength alongside their suffering. One of the biggest barriers to vicarious resilience is pity. When you pity someone, you feel sorry for their suffering but do not see their strength, and you do not see yourself in their story. In many ways, pity is a safer emotion than genuine empathy. It lets you protect yourself from sharing too closely in someone else's distress. You can maintain the fiction that you will never suffer in that way. However, in addition to diminishing the person who is the object of your pity, it also blocks your capacity to experience vicarious growth. The process of learning and growing from another person's suffering seems to require being affected by that suffering. It is not about passively witnessing resilience in another. It is about allowing yourself to be touched by their suffering and their strength.

One marriage and family therapist who worked with survivors of torture reflected on how vicarious resilience requires a radical mindset shift about how to relate to a client's suffering:

We often think about vicarious trauma as being a kind of radiation that someone's infected with . . . and it leaks out to us, and we have to have barriers, and we have to cleanse ourselves, and all these metaphors. But you can think of vicarious resilience as being more like a flow of energy. . . . It just flows out of them, this kind of love or hope or pure energy that's this life force. And so you get infected or affected by that as well.

Research shows that simply bringing attention to the concept of vicarious resilience makes that response more likely—just as telling people about post-traumatic growth increases the chance that they will experience it themselves. Even now, having read these pages, you are more likely to be strengthened by the suffering and growth of others. When you find yourself in the presence of another person's suffering, try to be a witness to both their pain and their resources. Let yourself by touched by their experience, but also awed by their resilience.

TELLING STORIES THAT INSPIRE RESILIENCE

When a patient walks the halls at St. Jude Children's Research Hospital in Memphis, Tennessee, one thing they'll see is the wall of hope. The wall is lined with framed photographs of adults holding photographs of themselves as children. Every one of them is a survivor of childhood cancer or another life-threatening condition. The childhood photos date back to their treatment days at St. Jude. In those early photos, some are bald from chemotherapy. Others pose with their doctors or parents. The adults holding those photos are proof that healing is possible. Even more incredibly, half of them now work at St. Jude as doctors, nurses, or researchers. They transformed tragedy into purpose, and returned to St. Jude to give back to the community that helped them.

There are many ways to tell stories of resilience and growth. Sometimes the storytelling is through news reports, but sometimes it is through artwork, photographs, and other images. Sometimes it is through websites, letters, or one-on-one conversations. Any organization or community can choose to share stories of growth, connection, and resilience. Consider these examples:

- A newsletter for parents of middle schoolers reports on how employees donated sick days to a teacher battling breast cancer, along with the good news that the teacher is now in remission and back in the classroom.
- A company CEO decides to use a company-wide meeting to introduce the team that turned around a failing product.
- A church leader invites a community member to share with the congregation how she first came to the church in need of food and shelter and now volunteers in those same church programs to help others.
- A local coffee shop displays pictures of its staff helping to rebuild a community park damaged by a storm.
- A physical therapy center asks patients nearing the end of rehabilitation to write letters about their struggles and growth to encourage future patients.

These are the kinds of stories I noticed, when I started looking for them. Importantly, being exposed to such stories and images makes people more likely to experience growth from their own struggles. For example, in Queensland, Australia, 246 police recruits were randomly assigned to a special program called Promoting Resilient Officers, which introduced recruits to the idea that adversity can lead to growth. As part of the program, recruits watched a video of a senior officer discussing his twenty years of experience on the force. He shared what it was like to work on the sexual assault team and how his life had changed as a result of the traumatic experiences he had endured over the years. The stories were carefully chosen to demonstrate different aspects of post-traumatic growth, including a greater appreciation for life, a sense of personal strength, and spiritual growth.

The researchers hoped that hearing these stories of post-traumatic growth would help the new police recruits when they encountered traumatic events in the line of duty. Early results suggest it is working. Six months after they had participated in the program, new offi-

---

Transform Stress: Tell Your Own Story of Growth and Resilience

One of the best ways to notice, value, and express your own growth is to reflect on a difficult time in your life as if you were a journalist writing a restorative narrative. How would a storyteller describe the challenges you have faced? What would a good observer see as a turning point in your story— a moment when you were able to reengage or find meaning? If a journalist were to follow you for a week, what evidence would the journalist see of your strength and resilience? What do you do that demonstrates your growth or expresses your values? What would friends, family, coworkers, or others who have witnessed your journey say to describe how you have changed or grown? What objects in your home or office would a photojournalist want to photograph as evidence of your growth or resilience?

Consider taking some time to write your own story about any experience that you view as both stressful and a source of growth or meaning. Or use any medium that appeals to you, such as photo collage, drawing, or video. This exercise can be very personal or private, and you never need to share it with anyone. But it can also be a wonderful exercise to share with others.

cers who had experienced a trauma on the job or in their personal lives reported significantly higher post-traumatic growth than officers in a control group who did not go through the program.

We all tell stories, and the stories we choose to tell can create a culture of resilience. How do you tell the stories of your family? Your community? Your company? Your own life? Consider how you might make room for stories that reflect the strength, courage, compassion, and resilience in yourself and in your community.

Final Thoughts

Earlier in this book, I mentioned that after students take my New Science of Stress course, they are less likely to agree with the statement "If I could magically remove all the painful experiences I've had in my life, I would do so." They are also less likely to agree with the statement "My painful experiences and memories make it difficult for me to live a life that I would value." How do you feel when you think about these statements? Would you go back and remove all the painful experiences in your life?

How you answer that question matters. People who agree with statements like these are less satisfied with their current lives, more anxious about the future, and more likely to become depressed. These outcomes don't seem to be the direct result of a person's painful experiences, but rather the result of their attitude toward them. Importantly, it is possible to learn to think about your struggles in a different way. Studies show that when people adopt a more accepting attitude toward their past hardships, they become happier, less depressed, and more resilient.

Choosing to see the upside in our most painful experiences is part of how we can change our relationships with stress. Accepting past adversity is part of how we find the courage to grow from our present struggles. In many ways, it is the attitude that allows us to embrace and transform stress. And while I have shared with you some of the science that supports a growth mindset toward adversity, the evidence for this point of view is already all around you. If you look, you will see the signs of it in your own life, in the lives of those you admire, and even in the stories of strangers.

final reflections

F OR MOST OF its history, the science of stress focused on one question: Is stress bad for you? (Eventually, it graduated to the question, Just how bad is stress for you?)

But the interesting thing about the science of stress is that despite the overwhelmingly accepted idea that stress is harmful, the research tells a slightly different story: Stress is harmful, *except when it's not.* Consider the examples we've seen in this book: Stress increases the risk of health problems, except when people regularly give back to their communities. Stress increases the risk of dying, except when people have a sense of purpose. Stress increases the risk of depression, except when people see a benefit in their struggles. Stress is paralyzing, except when people perceive themselves as capable. Stress is debilitating, except when it helps you perform. Stress makes people selfish, except when it makes them altruistic. For every harmful outcome you can think of, there's an exception that erases the expected association between stress and something bad—and often replaces it with an unexpected benefit.

What makes these exceptions so interesting is that they are hardly exceptional at all. The things that protect us from the dreaded dangers of stress are all attainable. Think about the mindset exercises and strategies described in this book: Choosing to remember your most important values so that it is easier to find the meaning in everyday stress. Having open and honest conversations about your struggles so that you feel less alone in your suffering. Viewing your body's stress response as a resource so that you can trust yourself to handle the pressure and rise to the challenge. Going out of your way to help someone else so that you can access the biology of hope and courage. Not only are these strategies accessible, but they also don't require you to achieve the one thing that most people think they need to do, but that turns out to be an impossible and self-destructive goal: to avoid stress.

Rather than determining once and for all "Is stress bad?" or "Is stress good?", I am now most interested in understanding how the stance we take toward stress matters. A better question for each of us to ask ourselves, as individuals trying to cope with stress, might be: *Do I believe I have the capacity to transform stress into something good?* Mindsets are not black-and-white truths about the world. They are based on evidence, but they are also stances we choose to take toward life.

The science also tells us that stress is most likely to be harmful when three things are true:

1. You feel inadequate to it;
2. It isolates you from others; and
3. It feels utterly meaningless and against your will.

As we've seen, how you think about stress feeds into each one of these factors. When you view stress as inevitably harmful and something to avoid, you become more likely to feel all of these things: doubt about your ability to handle the challenges you face, alone in your suffering, and unable to find meaning in your struggles. In contrast, accepting and embracing stress can transform these states into a totally different experience. Self-doubt is replaced by confidence, fear becomes courage, isolation turns into connection, and suffering gives rise to meaning. And all without getting rid of the stress.

NOT LONG ago, I received an email from Jeremy Jamieson, the psychologist who studies how embracing anxiety can enhance performance. He wrote about how he has been rethinking another unpopular feeling lately: fatigue. Jamieson, at age thirty-three, now has a one-year-old at home. He wrote, "My wife and I were reflecting that feeling exhausted at the end of the day is a sign that we gave it our all."

This email made me smile because it was such a simple illustration of his stress mindset in action. He didn't view his physical state as a sign that something was wrong with him or his life, and that helped him see the meaning in one of the most stressful aspects of being a new dad. The email reminded me of similar thoughts I've had since I began to rethink stress. I now find myself almost effortlessly reappraising stress, even if I find myself first complaining out of habit, "This is so stressful!"

When I committed myself to the process of embracing stress, I didn't anticipate the biggest way it would affect my everyday experience of life. To my surprise, I started to feel a flood of gratitude in situations I would also describe as highly stressful. It wasn't an intentional mindset shift; the gratitude just showed up. I still haven't fully figured out why this was the biggest change for me, but it probably has something to do with what was most toxic about my experience of stress before I embraced it—a habit of resenting the things in my life that caused stress because I found the experience of stress so distressing.

I've observed that the effects of embracing stress seem to follow this pattern—changing exactly whatever is most toxic about the relationship each person has with the stress in his or her life. Students tell me about being less afraid, less lonely, or more enthusiastic about life. They feel less victimized by their lives, or less guilty for having a stressful life. Some are able to trust others more, others are able to stand up for themselves for the first time. Some find themselves feeling less angry about things that happened in their past and more hopeful about the future. My working hypothesis? That in each case, this is just what was needed to transform their experiences of stress.

When you put away this book, you likely won't have a clear sense yet of how its ideas will take root in your life. That's part of the magic of mindset interventions. If the science holds true, you might not even remember what this book was about. If I were to track you down a year from now and ask you what your favorite part was, would you remember the story of Selye's rats? Or think about the Sole Train runners cheering one another on? Would you still be rethinking your racing heart or trying to remember your bigger-than-self goals?

Or would you struggle to remember any of the details at all?

I can live with that. I trust that what you most needed to hear, you will remember—maybe not in the intellectual way of being able to repeat from memory any specific study or story, but in the way that new mindsets often land: in the heart, where they encourage you, inspire you, and change how you see yourself and the world.

So much of this book has been about telling stories that I want to end with one more.

A while back, one of my close friends shared with me that instead of New Year's resolutions, her family had started to set annual stress goals. Each year, she, her husband, and their teenage son decide how they want to grow in the coming year. Then they choose a personal project that will be both meaningful and difficult. They talk about what their stress edge will be—what they expect to be challenging, what they might feel anxious about, and the strengths that they want to develop.

I fell in love with this idea and immediately began using it myself. Not just for New Year's resolutions but as an orientation to life. In fact, writing this book was one of my big stress goals for the past two years. I knew it would be hard to do justice to the breadth of scientific research, and I was most worried about my ability to honor the incredible range of what people mean when they talk about stress. The strength I needed to develop was my willingness to keep asking people to tell me the truth about their experience of stress—even when it made writing the book more complicated, or forced me to live with questions I knew I couldn't neatly answer.

Now, because this book is a mindset intervention, you've probably already recognized that this story is also an invitation to set your own stress goal. Any new beginning or transition is an opportunity to think about how you want to challenge yourself. Birthdays, the start of a new calendar or school year, Sunday evenings, or each morning as you think about the day ahead. Even right now, you could ask yourself, "How do I want to grow from stress?" If there's one thing I've learned, it's that any moment can become a turning point in how you experience stress, if you choose to make it one.

acknowledgments

WRITING A BOOK is stressful—and I mean that in the good way. But I couldn't have done it without a lot of other people. Here's the history of this book in thank-yous:

You may have picked up this book because you saw a video of the talk I gave at TEDGlobal in Edinburgh in 2013. I had actually started working on a book about stress seven years before I gave the talk "How to Make Stress Your Friend." However, without the TED Talk experience, I would not have had the courage to write *this* book. So thank you to TED organizers Bruno Giussani and Chris Anderson for showing me that the world was ready to rethink stress. Special thanks also to my twin sister and TED Talk veteran, Jane McGonigal, who convinced me that giving a TED Talk was a good idea (it seemed kind of stressful . . .) and then convinced the TED organizers that they should put me on the big red dot.

To the entire team at Avery and Penguin Random House. It started when I sent a list of possible topics for my next book, and every-one immediately said the one you wanted was the one I was most terrified—I mean, excited—to write. So thank you for seeing the upside of stress before I'd written it. Special gratitude to Megan New-man, the editor of this book. What you most appreciated in the first draft of this manuscript also happened to be the elements that were most meaningful to me—and that gave me the confidence to keep them in. A big thanks to Brian Tart, William Shinker, and Lisa John-son, who have made Avery such a great home for me as an author and who believed in this book early on. Of course, you probably never would have heard of this book without Lindsay Gordon and Casey Maloney, a dream team in the world of book publicity. To everyone at Avery and Penguin Random House, I also appreciate all the vegan meals you ate in my honor.

If you read my last book's acknowledgments, you already know that I have the best literary agent in the world, Ted Weinstein. So if you are an author and you haven't sent him your proposal yet, all I can say is . . . why not? I also have an amazing team of international support, and I want to thank in particular Manami Tamaoki and the entire Tuttle-Mori Agency in Tokyo, Japan, for connecting me to an audience halfway around the world.

Next, a big thank-you to the researchers who emailed, called, Skyped, or met with me in person to help me understand their work, especially Miranda Beltzer, Steve Cole, Jennifer Crocker, Alia Crum, Jeremy Jamieson, Susan Loeb, Ashley Martin, Crystal Park, Michael Poulin, Jane Shakespeare-Finch, Martin Turner, Mark Seery, Greg Walton, Monica Worline, and David Yeager. My deep appreciation for your dedicating your lives to conducting science that both relieves suffering and increases meaning in other people's lives. If I got any-thing wrong in my attempts to translate the science to a broader audi-ence, please forgive me—and correct me.

Gratitude also to the program developers, directors, teachers, and other folks on the front lines whose work changes the lives of so many, and who spoke with me for this book: Aaron Altose of Cuyahoga Community College, Sue Cotter of the Community Services Agency in Modesto, Jessica Leffler and Natalie Stavas of Sole Train, Diana Adamson and Noel Ramirez of ScholarMatch, Lennon Flowers of the Dinner Party, Jennifer White of Hope After Project, Mallary Jean Tenore of Images and Voices of Hope, and Mary Wiltenburg of the *Christian Science Monitor*. It is a gift to be able to share your work and stories with readers.

Thank you to my students at Stanford, especially those who took my Continuing Studies course, the New Science of Stress. You thought you were going to get rid of your stress, but I told you were going to embrace it, and almost none of you dropped the course. Thanks for that, and for asking tough questions, and *especially* to those of you who so generously shared your stories for the book. Consider your mindset shift official.

It takes a village to get an author to stop procrastinating and actually finish a book, even if that author has previously written a book about willpower. So thank you to my three writing buddies—Leah Weiss Ekstrom, Marina Krakovsky, and Jane McGonigal—who checked in every now and then to make sure that I was doing something that might eventually result in an actual book. Thanks also to Connie Hale, whose helpful advice on my first draft made the results significantly more readable.

The biggest thank-you goes to my husband, Brian Kidd, who has been through the book-writing process with me three times now, and assures me it is getting less traumatic for him and the household each time. Hopefully, he caught some vicarious post-traumatic growth this round as well.

notes

Introduction

High levels of stress increased the risk . . . Keller, Abiola, Kristen Litzelman, Lauren E. Wisk, et al. (2011). "Does the Perception That Stress Affects Health Matter? The Association with Health and Mortality." *Health Psychology* 31, no. 5: 677–84.

Those who had a positive view of aging . . . Levy, Becca R., Martin D. Slade, Suzanne R. Kunkel, and Stanislav V. Kasl. "Longevity Increased by Positive Self-Perceptions of Aging." *Journal of Personality and Social Psychology* 83, no. 2 (2002): 261–70.

In contrast, 60 percent . . . Barefoot, John C., Kimberly E. Maynard, Jean C. Beckham, Beverly H. Brummett, Karen Hooker, and Ilene C. Siegler. "Trust, Health, and Longevity." *Journal of Behavioral Medicine* 21, no. 6 (1998): 517–26.

The most threatening images . . . Hansen, Jochim, Susanne Winzeler, and Sascha Topolinski. "When the Death Makes You Smoke: A Terror Management Perspective on the Effectiveness of Cigarette On-Pack Warnings." *Journal of Experimental Social Psychology* 46, no. 1 (2010): 226–28.

In one study at the University of California ... Major, Brenda, Jeffrey M. Hunger, Debra P. Bunyan, and Carol T. Miller. "The Ironic Effects of Weight Stigma." *Journal of Experimental Social Psychology* 51 (2014): 74–80.

And yet, when put to the scientific test ... Peters, Gjalt-Jorn Ygram, Robert A.C. Ruiter, and Gerjo Kok. "Threatening Communication: A Critical Re-Analysis and a Revised Meta-Analytic Test of Fear Appeal Theory." *Health Psychology Review* 7, sup. 1 (2013): S8–S31. Peters, Gjalt-Jorn Y., Robert A.C. Ruiter, and Gerjo Kok. "Threatening Communication: A Qualitative Study of Fear Appeal Effectiveness Beliefs Among Intervention Developers, Policymakers, Politicians, Scientists, and Advertising Professionals." *International Journal of Psychology* 49, no. 2 (2014): 71–79.

Chapter 1. How to Change Your Mind About Stress

"Thinking Away the Pounds" and "Believe Yourself Healthy" ... Crum, Alia J., and Ellen J. Langer. "Mind-Set Matters: Exercise and the Placebo Effect." *Psychological Science* 18, no. 2 (2007): 165–71.

Crum's next headline-making study ... Crum, Alia J., William R. Corbin, Kelly D. Brownell, and Peter Salovey. "Mind over Milkshakes: Mindsets, Not Just Nutrients, Determine Ghrelin Response." *Health Psychology* 30, no. 4 (2011): 424–29.

Crum's most recent study ... Crum, Alia J., Modupe Akinola, Ashley Martin, and Sean Fath. "Improving Stress Without Reducing Stress: The Benefits of a Stress Is Enhancing Mindset in Both Challenging and Threatening Contexts." Manuscript unpublished, in progress (2015). Data partially presented at: Martin, A.M., Alia J. Crum, and Modupe A. Akinola. "The Buffering Effects of Stress Mindset on Cognitive Functioning During Stress." Poster presented at the 2014 Society for Personality and Social Psychology Conference, Austin, Texas.

In contrast, higher levels of DHEA have . . . Boudarene, M., J.J. Legros, and M. Timsit-Berthier. "[Study of the Stress Response: Role of Anxiety, Cortisol, and DHEAs]." *L'Encephale* 28, no. 2 (2001): 139–46.

It predicts academic persistence . . . Wemm, Stephanie, Tiniza Koone, Eric R. Blough, Steven Mewaldt, and Massimo Bardi. "The Role of DHEA in Relation to Problem Solving and Academic Performance." *Biological Psychology* 85, no. 1 (2010): 53–61.

During military survival training . . . Morgan, Charles A., Steve Southwick, Gary Hazlett, Ann Rasmusson, Gary Hoyt, Zoran Zimolo, and Dennis Charney. "Relationships Among Plasma Dehydroepiandrosterone Sulfate and Cortisol Levels, Symptoms of Dissociation, and Objective Performance in Humans Exposed to Acute Stress." *Archives of General Psychiatry* 61, no. 8 (2004): 819–25. See also Rasmusson, Ann M., Meena Vythilingam, and Charles A. Morgan III. "The Neuroendocrinology of Posttraumatic Stress Disorder: New Directions." *CNS Spectrums* 8, no. 9 (2003): 651–67.

The growth index even predicts . . . Cicchetti, Dante, and Fred A. Rogosch. "Adaptive Coping Under Conditions of Extreme Stress: Multilevel Influences on the Determinants of Resilience in Maltreated Children." *New Directions for Child and Adolescent Development* 2009, no. 124 (2009): 47–59.

For an excellent introduction to the concept of mindsets, see Dweck, Carol. *Mindset: The New Psychology of Success*. Random House LLC, 2006.

For example, the Baltimore Longitudinal Study of Aging . . . Levy, Becca R., Alan B. Zonderman, Martin D. Slade, and Luigi Ferrucci. "Age Stereotypes Held Earlier in Life Predict Cardiovascular Events in Later Life." *Psychological Science* 20, no. 3 (2009): 296–98.

In one study, adults who . . . Levy, Becca R., Martin D. Slade,

Jeanine May, and Eugene A. Caracciolo. "Physical Recovery After Acute Myocardial Infarction: Positive Age Self-Stereotypes as a Resource." *International Journal of Aging and Human Development* 62, no. 4 (2006): 285–301.

In another study, a positive view . . . Levy, Becca R., Martin D. Slade, Terrence E. Murphy, and Thomas M. Gill. "Association Between Positive Age Stereotypes and Recovery from Disability in Older Persons." *JAMA* 308, no. 19 (2012): 1972–73.

By the way, if these findings . . . The work of Stanford psychologist Laura Carstensen demonstrates that people get happier as they grow older, among other psychological benefits of aging. For example, see Carstensen, Laura L., Bulent Turan, Susanne Scheibe, Nilam Ram, Hal Ersner-Hershfield, Gregory R. Samanez-Larkin, Kathryn P. Brooks, and John R. Nesselroade. "Emotional Experience Improves with Age: Evidence Based on Over 10 Years of Experience Sampling." *Psychology and Aging* 26, no. 1 (2011): 21–33.

For example, an intervention . . . Wolff, Julia K., Lisa M. Warner, Jochen P. Ziegelmann, and Susanne Wurm. "What Do Targeting Positive Views on Aging Add to a Physical Activity Intervention in Older Adults? Results from a Randomised Controlled Trial." *Psychology and Health* (ahead of print, 2014): 1–18.

Researchers at the German Centre . . . Wurm, Susanne, Lisa M. Warner, Jochen P. Ziegelmann, Julia K. Wolff, and Benjamin Schüz. "How Do Negative Self-Perceptions of Aging Become a Self-Fulfilling Prophecy?" *Psychology and Aging* 28, no. 4 (2013): 1088–97.

People who hold negative views of aging . . . Levy, Becca R., Martin D. Slade, Suzanne R. Kunkel, and Stanislav V. Kasl. "Longevity Increased by Positive Self-Perceptions of Aging." *Journal of Personality and Social Psychology* 83, no. 2 (2002): 261–70.

In contrast, those exposed to negative . . . Levy, Becca, Ori Ashman, and Itiel Dror. "To Be or Not to Be: The Effects of Aging Stereotypes on the Will to Live." *OMEGA Journal of Death and Dying* 40, no. 3 (2000): 409–20.

Take a moment to look . . . These items are taken from the Stress Mindset Measure, originally published in: Crum, Alia J., Peter Salovey, and Shawn Achor. "Rethinking Stress: The Role of Mindsets in Determining the Stress Response." *Journal of Personality and Social Psychology* 104, no. 4 (2013): 716–33. The Stress Mindset Measure is reproduced with permission. Copyright 2013 by the American Psychological Association.

Men and women do not differ . . . Ibid.

In a 2014 survey conducted . . . The NPR/Robert Wood Johnson Foundation/Harvard School of Public Health Burden of Stress in America Survey was conducted from March 5 to April 8, 2014, with a sample of 2,505 respondents.

Even those who report relatively . . . The Stress in America survey is an annual survey within the United States conducted by Harris Interactive on behalf of the American Psychological Association. The full 2013 report was released by the American Psychological Association on February 11, 2014. http://www.apa.org/news/press/releases/stress/2013/stress-report.pdf.

And in the 2014 Harvard School . . . The NPR/Robert Wood Johnson Foundation/Harvard School of Public Health Burden of Stress in America Survey was conducted from March 5 to April 8, 2014, with a sample of 2,505 respondents.

People who endorse a stress-is-harmful mindset are more likely to say that they cope with stress . . . Crum, Alia. "Rethinking Stress: The Role of Mindsets in Determining the Stress Response." PhD dissertation, Yale University, 2012.

One study found that within ten years . . . Michel, Alexandra. "Transcending Socialization: A Nine-Year Ethnography of the

Body's Role in Organizational Control and Knowledge Workers' Transformation." *Administrative Science Quarterly* 56, no. 3 (2012): 325–68.

Financial workers reported significantly . . . Tsai, Feng-Jen, and Chang-Chuan Chan. "The Impact of the 2008 Financial Crisis on Psychological Work Stress Among Financial Workers and Lawyers." *International Archives of Occupational and Environmental Health* 84, no. 4 (2011): 445–52.

Across the industry, there were widespread reports . . . John Aidan Byrne. "The Casualties of Wall Street." WealthManagement.com. June 1, 2009. http://wealthmanagement.com/practice-management /casualties-wall-street. Accessed August 9, 2014.

UBS instituted major layoffs . . . UBS Annual Report 2008. Available at http://www.ubs.com/global/en/about_ubs/investor _relations/restatement.html. Accessed August 10, 2014.

The employees were randomly assigned . . . Crum, Alia, Peter Salovey, and Shawn Achor. "Evaluating a Mindset Training Program to Unleash the Enhancing Nature of Stress." *Academy of Management Proceedings*, vol. 2011, no. 1: 1–6.

Then he follows people over time . . . For an introduction to brief mindset interventions, see Walton, Gregory M. "The New Science of Wise Psychological Interventions." *Current Directions in Psychological Science* 23, no. 1 (2014): 73–82.

When I asked Walton what his favorite . . . Walton, Gregory M., and Geoffrey L. Cohen. "A Brief Social-Belonging Intervention Improves Academic and Health Outcomes of Minority Students." *Science* 331, no. 6023 (2011): 1447–51. Personal interview conducted with Greg Walton on February 20, 2014.

Walton and his colleagues have delivered . . . Yeager, David S., and Gregory M. Walton. "Social-Psychological Interventions in Education: They're Not Magic." *Review of Educational Research* 81, no. 2 (2011): 267–301. Yeager, David S., Dave Paunesku, Gregory

M. Walton, and Carol S. Dweck. "How Can We Instill Productive Mindsets at Scale? A Review of the Evidence and an Initial R&D Agenda." White paper prepared for the White House meeting "Excellence in Education: The Importance of Academic Mindsets." May 10, 2013.

"Their social world is changing" . . . Walton, Gregory M., Christine Logel, Jennifer M. Peach, Steven J. Spencer, and Mark P. Zanna. "Two Brief Interventions to Mitigate a 'Chilly Climate' Transform Women's Experience, Relationships, and Achievement in Engineering." (2014, in press.)

Despite the staff member's pessimism . . . Yeager, David Scott, Rebecca Johnson, Brian James Spitzer, Kali H. Trzesniewski, Joseph Powers, and Carol S. Dweck. "The Far-Reaching Effects of Believing People Can Change: Implicit Theories of Personality Shape Stress, Health, and Achievement During Adolescence." *Journal of Personality and Social Psychology* 106, no. 6 (2014): 867–81. See also Miu, Adriana Sum, David Scott Yeager, David Sherman, James Pennebaker, and Kali Trzesniewski. "Preventing Depression by Teaching Adolescents That People Can Change: Nine-Month Effects of a Brief Incremental Theory of Personality Intervention." (2014, in press.) Some details from a personal interview conducted with David Yeager, May 23, 2014.

Surprisingly, pills clearly labeled . . . Kelley, John M., Ted J. Kaptchuk, Cristina Cusin, Samuel Lipkin, and Maurizio Fava. "Open-Label Placebo for Major Depressive Disorder: A Pilot Randomized Controlled Trial." *Psychotherapy and Psychosomatics* 81, no. 5 (2012): 312–14. See also Kam-Hansen, Slavenka, Moshe Jakubowski, John M. Kelley, Irving Kirsch, David C. Hoaglin, Ted J. Kaptchuk, and Rami Burstein. "Altered Placebo and Drug Labeling Changes the Outcome of Episodic Migraine Attacks." *Science Translational Medicine* 6, no. 218 (2014): 218ra5–218ra5.

When people are told how . . . Silverman, Arielle, Christine Logel, and Geoffrey L. Cohen. "Self-Affirmation as a Deliberate Coping Strategy: The Moderating Role of Choice." *Journal of Experimental Social Psychology* 49, no. 1 (2013): 93–98. Cohen, Geoffrey L., and David K. Sherman. "The Psychology of Change: Self-Affirmation and Social Psychological Intervention." *Annual Review of Psychology* 65 (2014): 333–71.

Chapter 2. Beyond Fight-Or-Flight

In the late 1990s, an unusual . . . Delahanty, Douglas L., A. Jay Raimonde, and Eileen Spoonster. "Initial Posttraumatic Urinary Cortisol Levels Predict Subsequent PTSD Symptoms in Motor Vehicle Accident Victims." *Biological Psychiatry* 48, no. 9 (2000): 940–47. See also Walsh, Kate, Nicole R. Nugent, Amelia Kotte, Ananda B. Amstadter, Sheila Wang, Constance Guille, Ron Acierno, Dean G. Kilpatrick, and Heidi S. Resnick. "Cortisol at the Emergency Room Rape Visit as a Predictor of PTSD and Depression Symptoms over Time." *Psychoneuroendocrinology* 38, no. 11 (2013): 2520–28. Delahanty, Douglas L., Crystal Gabert-Quillen, Sarah A. Ostrowski, Nicole R. Nugent, Beth Fischer, Adam Morris, Roger K. Pitman, John Bon, and William Fallon. "The Efficacy of Initial Hydrocortisone Administration at Preventing Posttraumatic Distress in Adult Trauma Patients: A Randomized Trial." *CNS Spectrums* 18, no. 2 (2013): 103–11. Ehring, Thomas, Anke Ehlers, Anthony J. Cleare, and Edward Glucksman. "Do Acute Psychological and Psychobiological Responses to Trauma Predict Subsequent Symptom Severities of PTSD and Depression?" *Psychiatry Research* 161, no. 1 (2008): 67–75.

In fact, one of the most . . . de Quervain, Dominique J-F., Dorothée Bentz, Tanja Michael, Olivia C. Bolt, Brenda K. Wiederhold, Jürgen Margraf, and Frank H. Wilhelm. "Glucocorticoids Enhance Extinction-Based Psychotherapy." *Proceedings of the National Academy of Sciences* 108, no. 16 (2011): 6621–25. de Quervain, Dominique J-F., and Jürgen Margraf. "Glucocorticoids for the Treatment of Post-Traumatic Stress Disorder and Phobias: A Novel Therapeutic Approach." *European Journal of Pharmacology* 583, no. 2 (2008): 365–71.

After taking ten milligrams of cortisol . . . Aerni, Amanda, Rafael Traber, Christoph Hock, Benno Roozendaal, Gustav Schelling, Andreas Papassotiropoulos, Roger M. Nitsch, Ulrich Schnyder, and J-F. Dominique. "Low-Dose Cortisol for Symptoms of Posttraumatic Stress Disorder." *American Journal of Psychiatry* 161, no. 8 (2004): 1488–90.

Among high-risk cardiac surgery patients . . . Weis, Florian, Erich Kilger, Benno Roozendaal, Dominique J-F. de Quervain, Peter Lamm, Michael Schmidt, Martin Schmölz, Josef Briegel, and Gustav Schelling. "Stress Doses of Hydrocortisone Reduce Chronic Stress Symptoms and Improve Health-Related Quality of Life in High-Risk Patients After Cardiac Surgery: A Randomized Study." *Journal of Thoracic and Cardiovascular Surgery* 131, no. 2 (2006): 277–82. Schelling, Gustav, Benno Roozendaal, Till Krauseneck, Martin Schmoelz, Dominique J-F. de Quervain, and Josef Briegel. "Efficacy of Hydrocortisone in Preventing Posttraumatic Stress Disorder Following Critical Illness and Major Surgery." *Annals of the New York Academy of Sciences* 1071, no. 1 (2006): 46–53.

Taking a dose of stress hormones . . . Bentz, Dorothée, Tanja Michael, Dominique J-F. de Quervain, and Frank H. Wilhelm. "Enhancing Exposure Therapy for Anxiety Disorders with Glucocorticoids: From Basic Mechanisms of Emotional Learning to Clinical Applications." *Journal of Anxiety Disorders* 24, no. 2 (2010): 223–230.

The year was 1936, and Hungarian endocrinologist Hans Selye . . . Selye, Hans. *The Stress of Life.* McGraw Hill, 1956. See also Selye, Hans. *The Stress of My Life: A Scientist's Memoirs.*

McClelland and Stewart Toronto, 1977. Selye, Hans. *Stress Without Distress*. Springer U.S., 1976.

The tobacco industry paid him . . . Petticrew, Mark P., and Kelley Lee. "The 'Father of Stress' Meets 'Big Tobacco': Hans Selye and the Tobacco Industry." *American Journal of Public Health* 101, no. 3 (2011): 411–18.

He even tried to improve stress's image . . . Selye's quote "There is always stress . . ." is taken from an interview published in Oates Jr., Robert M. *Celebrating the Dawn: Maharishi Mahesh Yogi and the TM Technique*. New York: G.P. Putnam's Sons, 1976.

For some perspective, consider that in a major 2014 survey . . . The NPR/Robert Wood Johnson Foundation/Harvard School of Public Health Burden of Stress in America Survey was conducted from March 5 to April 8, 2014, with a sample of 2,505 respondents.

A 2011 review of over a hundred studies . . . Schetter, Christine. "Psychological Science on Pregnancy: Stress Processes, Biopsychosocial Models, and Emerging Research Issues." *Annual Review of Psychology* 62 (2011): 531–58.

The exposure to a mom's stress hormones . . . DiPietro, Janet A., Katie T. Kivlighan, Kathleen A. Costigan, Suzanne E. Rubin, Dorothy E. Shiffler, Janice L. Henderson, and Joseph P. Pillion. "Prenatal Antecedents of Newborn Neurological Maturation." *Child Development* 81, no. 1 (2010): 115–30.

As one woman told the researchers . . . Watt, Melissa H., Lisa A. Eaton, Karmel W. Choi, Jennifer Velloza, Seth C. Kalichman, Donald Skinner, and Kathleen J. Sikkema. "'It's Better for Me to Drink, at Least the Stress Is Going Away': Perspectives on Alcohol Use During Pregnancy Among South African Women Attending Drinking Establishments." *Social Science and Medicine* 116 (2014): 119–25.

Stanford biopsychologist Karen Parker . . . Lyons, David M.,

Karen J. Parker, and Alan F. Schatzberg. "Animal Models of Early Life Stress: Implications For Understanding Resilience." *Developmental Psychobiology* 52, no. 7 (2010): 616–24. See also Lyons, David M., and Karen J. Parker. "Stress Inoculation-Induced Indications of Resilience in Monkeys." *Journal of Traumatic Stress* 20, no. 4 (2007): 423–33. Parker, Karen J., Christine L. Buckmaster, Steven E. Lindley, Alan F. Schatzberg, and David M. Lyons. "Hypothalamic-Pituitary-Adrenal Axis Physiology and Cognitive Control of Behavior in Stress Inoculated Monkeys." *International Journal of Behavioral Development* 36, no. 1 (2012): 45–52.

His favorite methods for making his animals angry . . . Cannon, Walter Bradford. *Bodily Changes in Pain, Hunger, Fear, and Rage: An Account of Recent Researches into the Function of Emotional Excitement.* D. Appleton and Company, 1915. The quote about a cat's breathing is on page 15.

It will also help you engage with challenges . . . Everly Jr., George S., and Jeffrey M. Lating. "The Anatomy and Physiology of the Human Stress Response." In *A Clinical Guide to the Treatment of the Human Stress Response*, edited by George S. Everly Jr. and Jeffrey M. Lating, 17–51. New York: Springer, 2013.

He considered this percentage . . . Van den Assem, Martijn J., Dennie Van Dolder, and Richard H. Thaler. "Split or Steal? Cooperative Behavior When the Stakes Are Large." *Management Science* 58, no. 1 (2012): 2–20.

In one study, men were put through . . . von Dawans, Bernadette, Urs Fischbacher, Clemens Kirschbaum, Ernst Fehr, and Markus Heinrichs. "The Social Dimension of Stress Reactivity: Acute Stress Increases Prosocial Behavior in Humans." *Psychological Science* 23, no. 6 (2012): 651–60.

Unlike what most people believe . . . Kemeny, Margaret E. "The Psychobiology of Stress." *Current Directions in Psychological Science* 12, no. 4 (2003): 124–29. See also Dickerson, Sally S., Tara

L. Gruenewald, and Margaret E. Kemeny. "When the Social Self Is Threatened: Shame, Physiology, and Health." *Journal of Personality* 72, no. 6 (2004): 1191–216.

"I don't know how I lifted it" . . . Fox News/Associated Press. "Oregon Man Pinned Under 3,000-Pound Tractor Saved by Teen Daughters." April 11, 2013. http://www.foxnews.com/us/2013/04 /11/oregon-man-pinned-under-3000-pound-tractor-saved-by-two -teen-daughters.

It's been observed both in skydivers . . . Allison, Amber L., Jeremy C. Peres, Christian Boettger, Uwe Leonbacher, Paul D. Hastings, and Elizabeth A. Shirtcliff. "Fight, Flight, or Fall: Autonomic Nervous System Reactivity During Skydiving." *Personality and Individual Differences* 53, no. 3 (2012): 218–23.

But when the stressful situation . . . Seery, Mark D. "The Biopsychosocial Model of Challenge and Threat: Using the Heart to Measure the Mind." *Social and Personality Psychology Compass* 7, no. 9 (2013): 637–53.

People who report being in a flow state . . . Peifer, Corinna. "Psychophysiological Correlates of Flow-Experience." *Advances in Flow Research*, edited by Stephan Engeser, 139–64. New York: Springer, 2012.

Scientists refer to this as . . . Taylor, Shelley E. "Tend and Befriend: Biobehavioral Bases of Affiliation Under Stress." *Current Directions in Psychological Science* 15, no. 6 (2006): 273–77. Buchanan, Tony W., and Stephanie D. Preston. "Stress Leads to Prosocial Action in Immediate Need Situations." *Frontiers in Behavioral Neuroscience* 8, no. 5 (2014): 1–6.

When researchers gave the rats a drug . . . Moghimian, Maryam, Mahdieh Faghihi, Seyed Morteza Karimian, Alireza Imani, Fariba Houshmand, and Yaser Azizi. "The Role of Central Oxytocin in Stress-Induced Cardioprotection in Ischemic-Reperfused Heart Model." *Journal of Cardiology* 61, no. 1 (2013): 79–86.

For example, cortisol and oxytocin . . . Laurent, Heidemarie K., Sean M. Laurent, and Douglas A. Granger. "Salivary Nerve Growth Factor Response to Stress Related to Resilience." *Physiology and Behavior* 129 (2014): 130–34.

People who release higher levels . . . Het, Serkan, Daniela Schoofs, Nicolas Rohleder, and Oliver T. Wolf. "Stress-Induced Cortisol Level Elevations Are Associated with Reduced Negative Affect After Stress: Indications for a Mood-Buffering Cortisol Effect." *Psychosomatic Medicine* 74, no. 1 (2012): 23–32. Walsh, Kate, Nicole R. Nugent, Amelia Kotte, Ananda B. Amstadter, Sheila Wang, Constance Guille, Ron Acierno, Dean G. Kilpatrick, and Heidi S. Resnick. "Cortisol at the Emergency Room Rape Visit as a Predictor of PTSD and Depression Symptoms Over Time." *Psychoneuroendocrinology* 38, no. 11 (2013): 2520–28.

Other studies show that viewing . . . Stout, Jane G., and Nilanjana Dasgupta. "Mastering One's Destiny: Mastery Goals Promote Challenge and Success Despite Social Identity Threat." *Personality and Social Psychology Bulletin* 39, no. 6 (2013): 748–62.

Your life history can also influence how you respond to stress . . . Pierrehumbert, Blaise, Raffaella Torrisi, Daniel Laufer, Oliver Halfon, François Ansermet, and M. Beck Popovic. "Oxytocin Response to an Experimental Psychosocial Challenge in Adults Exposed to Traumatic Experiences During Childhood or Adolescence." *Neuroscience* 166, no. 1 (2010): 168–77.

Other people are naturally more . . . Belsky, Jay, and Michael Pluess. "Beyond Diathesis Stress: Differential Susceptibility to Environmental Influences." *Psychological Bulletin* 135, no. 6 (2009): 885–908. Pluess, Michael, and Jay Belsky. "Vantage Sensitivity: Individual Differences in Response to Positive Experiences." *Psychological Bulletin* 139, no. 4 (2013): 901–16.

It's important to recognize that these . . . Del Giudice, Marco, J. Benjamin Hinnant, Bruce J. Ellis, and Mona El-Sheikh. "Adaptive

Patterns of Stress Responsivity: A Preliminary Investigation." *Developmental Psychology* 48, no. 3 (2012): 775–90. Del Giudice, Marco. "Early Stress and Human Behavioral Development: Emerging Evolutionary Perspectives." *Journal of Developmental Origins of Health and Disease* 5, no. 5 (2014): 270–80.

Chapter 3. A Meaningful Life Is a Stressful Life

From 2005 to 2006, researchers . . . Ng, Weiting, Ed Diener, Raksha Aurora, and James Harter. "Affluence, Feelings of Stress, and Well-Being." *Social Indicators Research* 94, no. 2 (2009): 257–71. Holmqvist, Goran, and Luisa Natali. "Exploring the Late Impact of the Great Recession Using Gallup World Poll Data." Innocenti Working Paper No. 2014-14. UNICEF Office of Research, Florence.

In contrast, the researchers . . . Tay, Louis, Ed Diener, Fritz Drasgow, and Jeroen K. Vermunt. "Multilevel Mixed-Measurement IRT Analysis: An Explication and Application to Self-Reported Emotions Across the World." *Organizational Research Methods* 14, no. 1 (2011): 177–207.

In 2013, researchers at . . . Baumeister, Roy F., Kathleen D. Vohs, Jennifer L. Aaker, and Emily N. Garbinsky. "Some Key Differences Between a Happy Life and a Meaningful Life." *Journal of Positive Psychology* 8, no. 6 (2013): 505–16.

When people report the biggest . . . The Stress in America survey is an annual survey within the United States conducted by Harris Interactive on behalf of the American Psychological Association. Full 2013 report released by the American Psychological Association on February 11, 2014.

In two recent surveys, 34 percent of adults . . . Kalms Annual Stress Report, a survey of two thousand men and women in the U.K. The survey results were released on November 4, 2013.

While 62 percent of highly stressed adults . . . Crompton, Susan. "What's Stressing the Stressed? Main Sources of Stress Among Workers." *Canadian Social Trends Component of Statistics Canada Catalogue no. 11-008-X.* Survey of 1,750 adults ages twenty to sixty-four. The findings were released October 13, 2011.

For example, the Gallup World Poll . . . Data on caring for kids comes from interviews with 131,159 adults in the United States conducted between January 2, 2014, and September 25, 2014, as part of the Gallup-Healthways Well-Being Index. See http://www.gallup.com/poll/178631/adults-children-home-greater-joy-stress.aspx. Data on entrepreneurs come from interviews with 273,175 adults in the United States conducted between January 2, 2011, and September 30, 2012. See http://www.gallup.com/poll/159131/entrepreneurship-comes-stress-optimism.aspx.

Although most people predict . . . Hsee, Christopher K., Adelle X. Yang, and Liangyan Wang. "Idleness Aversion and the Need for Justifiable Busyness." *Psychological Science* 21, no. 7 (2010): 926–30.

A dramatic *decrease* in busyness may . . . Sahlgren, Gabriel H. "Work Longer, Live Healthier: The Relationship Between Economic Activity, Health and Government Policy." Institute for Economic Affairs Discussion Paper, May 16, 2013.

In one large epidemiological study . . . Britton, Annie, and Martin J. Shipley. "Bored to Death?" *International Journal of Epidemiology* 39, no. 2 (2010): 370–71.

In contrast, many studies . . . Hill, Patrick L., and Nicholas A. Turiano. "Purpose in Life as a Predictor of Mortality Across Adulthood." *Psychological Science*, no. 25 (2014): 1482–86. See also Boyle, Patricia A., Lisa L. Barnes, Aron S. Buchman, and David A. Bennett. "Purpose in Life Is Associated with Mortality Among Community-Dwelling Older Persons." *Psychosomatic Medicine* 71, no. 5

(2009): 574–79. Krause, Neal. "Meaning in Life and Mortality." *Journals of Gerontology Series B: Psychological Sciences and Social Sciences* 64, no. 4 (2009): 517–27.

This reduced risk held even after controlling . . . Steptoe, Andrew, Angus Deaton, and Arthur A. Stone. "Subjective Wellbeing, Health, and Ageing." *Lancet* (2014, in press). doi: 10.1016/S0140-6736(13)61489-0.

A major study was released in 2014 . . . Aldwin, Carolyn M., Yu-Jin Jeong, Heidi Igarashi, Soyoung Choun, and Avron Spiro. "Do Hassles Mediate Between Life Events and Mortality in Older Men?: Longitudinal Findings from the VA Normative Aging Study." *Experimental Gerontology* 59 (2014): 74–80.

Feeling burdened rather than uplifted . . . Hazel, Nicholas A., and Benjamin L. Hankin. "A Trait-State-Error Model of Adult Hassles over Two Years: Magnitude, Sources, and Predictors of Stress Continuity." *Journal of Social and Clinical Psychology* 33, no. 2 (2014): 103–23.

The positive effect of writing . . . Keough, Kelli A., and Hazel Rose Markus. "The Role of the Self in Building the Bridge from Philosophy to Biology." *Psychological Inquiry* 9, no. 1 (1998): 49–53.

It turns out that writing about . . . Cohen, Geoffrey L., and David K. Sherman. "The Psychology of Change: Self-Affirmation and Social Psychological Intervention." *Annual Review of Psychology* 65 (2014): 333–71.

Reduces unhelpful rumination after a stressful experience . . . Koole, Sander L., Karianne Smeets, Ad Van Knippenberg, and Ap Dijksterhuis. "The Cessation of Rumination Through Self-Affirmation." *Journal of Personality and Social Psychology* 77, no. 1 (1999): 111–25.

It helps people persevere . . . reduces self-handicapping . . . Sherman, David K., Kimberly A. Hartson, Kevin R. Binning, Valerie Purdie-Vaughns, Julio Garcia, Suzanne Taborsky-Barba,

Sarah Tomassetti, A. David Nussbaum, and Geoffrey L. Cohen. "Deflecting the Trajectory and Changing the Narrative: How Self-Affirmation Affects Academic Performance and Motivation Under Identity Threat." *Journal of Personality and Social Psychology* 104, no. 4 (2013): 591–618. Siegel, Phyllis A., Joanne Scillitoe, and Rochelle Parks-Yancy. "Reducing the Tendency to Self-Handicap: The Effect of Self-Affirmation." *Journal of Experimental Social Psychology* 41, no. 6 (2005): 589–97.

In a study at the University of Waterloo . . . another version of this study . . . Fotuhi, Omid. "Implicit Processes in Smoking Interventions." A thesis presented to the University of Waterloo in fulfillment of the requirements for the PhD degree. Walton, Gregory M., Christine Logel, Jennifer M. Peach, Steven J. Spencer, and Mark P. Zanna. "Two Brief Interventions to Mitigate a 'Chilly Climate' Transform Women's Experience, Relationships, and Achievement in Engineering." *Journal of Educational Psychology* (2014, in press).

At the end of the program . . . Krasner, Michael S., Ronald M. Epstein, Howard Beckman, Anthony L. Suchman, Benjamin Chapman, Christopher J. Mooney, and Timothy E. Quill. "Association of an Educational Program in Mindful Communication with Burnout, Empathy, and Attitudes Among Primary Care Physicians." *JAMA* 302, no. 12 (2009): 1284–93. Details about the intervention were also sourced from facilitator training materials provided by the program creators.

As one reflected, "That feeling . . ." Physician quote from interviews reported in Beckman, Howard B., Melissa Wendland, Christopher Mooney, Michael S. Krasner, Timothy E. Quill, Anthony L. Suchman, and Ronald M. Epstein. "The Impact of a Program in Mindful Communication on Primary Care Physicians." *Academic Medicine* 87, no. 6 (2012): 815–19.

Psychologists have found that trying . . . Elliot, Andrew J.,

Constantine Sedikides, Kou Murayama, Ayumi Tanaka, Todd M. Thrash, and Rachel R. Mapes. "Cross-Cultural Generality and Specificity in Self-Regulation: Avoidance of Personal Goals and Multiple Aspects of Well-Being in the United States and Japan." *Emotion* 12, no. 5 (2012): 1031–40.

In a study of students at Doshisha University in Japan . . . Ibid.

For example, researchers at . . . Oertig, Daniela, Julia Schüler, Jessica Schnelle, Veronika Brandstätter, Marieke Roskes, and Andrew J. Elliot. "Avoidance of Goal Pursuit Depletes Self-Regulatory Resources." *Journal of Personality* 81, no. 4 (2013): 365–75.

Wherever a participant started in life . . . Holahan, Charles J., Rudolf H. Moos, Carole K. Holahan, Penny L. Brennan, and Kathleen K. Schutte. "Stress Generation, Avoidance Coping, and Depressive Symptoms: A 10-year model." *Journal of Consulting and Clinical Psychology* 73, no. 4 (2005): 658–66.

As psychologists Richard Ryan, Veronika Huta . . . Richard M., Veronika Huta, and Edward L. Deci. "Living Well: A Self-Determination Theory Perspective on Eudaimonia." *The Exploration of Happiness*, 117–39. Springer Netherlands, 2013.

As Maddi recalls . . . Maddi, Salvatore R. "The Story of Hardiness: Twenty Years of Theorizing, Research, and Practice." *Consulting Psychology Journal: Practice and Research* 54, no. 3 (2002): 173–85. Quote appears on page 174.

Maddi named this collection of attitudes . . . Maddi, Salvatore R. "On Hardiness and Other Pathways to Resilience." *American Psychologist* 60, no. 3 (2005): 261–62. Maddi, Salvatore R. "The Courage and Strategies of Hardiness as Helpful in Growing Despite Major, Disruptive Stresses." *American Psychologist* 63, no. 6 (2008): 563–64. Kobasa, Suzanne C., Salvatore R. Maddi, and Stephen Kahn. "Hardiness and Health: A Prospective Study." *Journal of Personality and Social Psychology* 42, no. 1 (1982): 168–77.

"When people think of child soldiers" . . . Quote originally appeared in Drexer, Madeline. "Life After Death: Helping Former Child Soldiers Become Whole Again." *Harvard Public Health Review,* Fall 2011: 18–25.

Betancourt has since conducted field . . . Ibid. Betancourt, Theresa S., Stephanie Simmons, Ivelina Borisova, Stephanie E. Brewer, Uzo Iweala, and Marie de la Soudière. "High Hopes, Grim Reality: Reintegration and the Education of Former Child Soldiers in Sierra Leone." *Comparative Education Review* 52, no. 4 (2008): 565–87. Betancourt, Theresa S., Robert T. Brennan, Julia Rubin-Smith, Garrett M. Fitzmaurice, and Stephen E. Gilman. "Sierra Leone's Former Child Soldiers: A Longitudinal Study of Risk, Protective Factors, and Mental Health." *Journal of the American Academy of Child and Adolescent Psychiatry* 49, no. 6 (2010): 606–15. Betancourt, Theresa Stichick, Sarah Meyers-Ohki, Sara N. Stulac, Amy Elizabeth Barrera, Christina Mushashi, and William R. Beardslee. "Nothing Can Defeat Combined Hands (*Abashize hamwe ntakibananira*): Protective Processes and Resilience in Rwandan Children and Families Affected by HIV/AIDS." *Social Science and Medicine* 73, no. 5 (2011): 693–701.

Chapter 4. Engage: How Anxiety Helps You Rise to the Challenge

Brooks designed an experiment . . . Brooks, Alison Wood. "Get Excited: Reappraising Pre-Performance Anxiety as Excitement." *Journal of Experimental Psychology: General* 143, no. 3 (2014): 1144–58.

Students who have greater increases in adrenaline . . . Dienstbier, Richard A. "Arousal and Physiological Toughness: Implications for Mental and Physical Health." *Psychological Review* 96, no. 1 (1989): 84–100.

Green Berets, Rangers, and Marines who . . . Morgan, Charles A.,

Sheila Wang, Ann Rasmusson, Gary Hazlett, George Anderson, and Dennis S. Charney. "Relationship Among Plasma Cortisol, Catecholamines, Neuropeptide Y, and Human Performance During Exposure to Uncontrollable Stress." *Psychosomatic Medicine* 63, no. 3 (2001): 412–22.

Federal law enforcement officers . . . Meyerhoff, James L., William Norris, George A. Saviolakis, Terry Wollert, Bob Burge, Valerie Atkins, and Charles Spielberger. "Evaluating Performance of Law Enforcement Personnel During a Stressful Training Scenario." *Annals of the New York Academy of Sciences* 1032, no. 1 (2004): 250–53.

People think that feeling . . . Jamieson, Jeremy P., Wendy Berry Mendes, Erin Blackstock, and Toni Schmader. "Turning the Knots in Your Stomach into Bows: Reappraising Arousal Improves Performance on the GRE." *Journal of Experimental Social Psychology* 46, no. 1 (2010): 208–12.

At the University of Lisbon . . . Strack, Juliane, and Francisco Esteves. "Exams? Why Worry? The Relationship Between Interpreting Anxiety as Facilitative, Stress Appraisals, Emotional Exhaustion, and Academic Performance." *Anxiety, Stress, and Coping: An International Journal* (2014): 1–10. doi: 10.1080/10615806.2014 .931942.

Researchers at Jacobs University . . . Strack, Juliane, Paulo N. Lopes, and Francisco Esteves. "Will You Thrive Under Pressure or Burn Out? Linking Anxiety Motivation and Emotional Exhaustion." *Cognition and Emotion.* Published electronically June 3, 2014: 1–14. doi: 10.1080/02699931.2014.922934.

The more pumped they were to take . . . Allison, Amber L., Jeremy C. Peres, Christian Boettger, Uwe Leonbacher, Paul D. Hastings, and Elizabeth A. Shirtcliff. "Fight, Flight, or Fall: Autonomic Nervous System Reactivity During Skydiving." *Personality and Individual Differences* 53, no. 3 (2012): 218–23.

Compared with only 25 percent . . . Adelson, Rachel. "Nervous About Numbers: Brain Patterns Reflect Math Anxiety." *Association for Psychological Science Observer* 27, no. 7 (2014): 35–37.

What matters is that the message . . . McKay, Brad, Rebecca Lewthwaite, and Gabriele Wulf. "Enhanced Expectancies Improve Performance Under Pressure." *Frontiers in Psychology* 3 (2012): 1–5.

Altose has seen the confidence that students . . . Information on the Cuyahoga Community College stress mindset intervention is from interviews and personal conversations with Aaron Altose and Jeremy Jamieson. For more information about the Achieving the Dream Network, see http://achievingthedream.org. For more information about the Carnegie Foundation for the Advancement of Teaching and the Alpha Lab Research Network, see http://commons.carnegiefoundation.org.

Middle-aged and older men . . . Yancura, Loriena A., Carolyn M. Aldwin, Michael R. Levenson, and Avron Spiro. "Coping, Affect, and the Metabolic Syndrome in Older Men: How Does Coping Get Under the Skin?" *Journals of Gerontology Series B: Psychological Sciences and Social Sciences* 61, no. 5 (2006): P295–P303.

And in the Framingham Heart Study . . . Jefferson, Angela L., Jayandra J. Himali, Alexa S. Beiser, Rhoda Au, Joseph M. Massaro, Sudha Seshadri, Philimon Gona, et al. "Cardiac Index Is Associated with Brain Aging: The Framingham Heart Study." *Circulation* 122, no. 7 (2010): 690–97.

During business negotiations, a challenge . . . de Wit, Frank R.C., Karen A. Jehn, and Daan Scheepers. "Negotiating Within Groups: A Psychophysiological Approach." *Research on Managing Groups and Teams* 14 (2011): 207–38.

Students with a challenge response . . . Seery, Mark D., Max Weisbuch, Maria A. Hetenyi, and Jim Blascovich. "Cardiovascular Measures Independently Predict Performance in a University Course." *Psychophysiology* 47, no. 3 (2010): 535–39. Turner, Martin J., Marc V.

Jones, David Sheffield, and Sophie L. Cross. "Cardiovascular Indices of Challenge and Threat States Predict Competitive Performance." *International Journal of Psychophysiology* 86, no. 1 (2012): 48–57.

Surgeons show better focus . . . Vine, Samuel J., Paul Freeman, Lee J. Moore, Roy Chandra-Ramanan, and Mark R. Wilson. "Evaluating Stress as a Challenge Is Associated with Superior Attentional Control and Motor Skill Performance: Testing the Predictions of the Biopsychosocial Model of Challenge and Threat." *Journal of Experimental Psychology: Applied* 19, no. 3 (2013): 185–94.

When faced with engine failure . . . Vine, Samuel J., Liis Uiga, Aureliu Lavric, Lee J. Moore, Krasimira Tsaneva-Atanasova, and Mark R. Wilson. "Individual Reactions to Stress Predict Performance During a Critical Aviation Incident." *Anxiety, Stress, and Coping.* (Ahead of print, 2014): 1–22.

Even what you learn from . . . van Wingen, Guido A., Elbert Geuze, Eric Vermetten, and Guillén Fernández. "Perceived Threat Predicts the Neural Sequelae of Combat Stress." *Molecular Psychiatry* 16, no. 6 (2011): 664–71.

These are all quick mindset shifts . . . Shnabel, Nurit, Valerie Purdie-Vaughns, Jonathan E. Cook, Julio Garcia, and Geoffrey L. Cohen. "Demystifying Values-Affirmation Interventions: Writing About Social Belonging Is a Key to Buffering Against Identity Threat." *Personality and Social Psychology Bulletin* 39, no. 5 (2013): 663–76. Cooper, Denise C., Julian F. Thayer, and Shari R. Waldstein. "Coping with Racism: The Impact of Prayer on Cardiovascular Reactivity and Post-Stress Recovery in African American Women." *Annals of Behavioral Medicine* 47, no. 2 (2014): 218–30. Krause, Neal. "The Perceived Prayers of Others, Stress, and Change in Depressive Symptoms over Time." *Review of Religious Research* 53, no. 3 (2011): 341–56.

Ever since it was developed . . . Allen, Andrew P., Paul J. Kennedy,

John F. Cryan, Timothy G. Dinan, and Gerard Clarke. "Biological and Psychological Markers of Stress in Humans: Focus on the Trier Social Stress Test." *Neuroscience and Biobehavioral Reviews* 38 (2014): 94–124.

One study found that when people . . . Lyons, Ian M., and Sian L. Beilock. "When Math Hurts: Math Anxiety Predicts Pain Network Activation in Anticipation of Doing Math." *PLOS ONE* 7, no. 10 (2012): e48076. See also Maloney, Erin A., Marjorie W. Schaeffer, and Sian L. Beilock. "Mathematics Anxiety and Stereotype Threat: Shared Mechanisms, Negative Consequences and Promising Interventions." *Research in Mathematics Education* 15, no. 2 (2013): 115–28.

Rethinking stress shifted their stress responses . . . Jamieson, Jeremy P., Matthew K. Nock, and Wendy Berry Mendes. "Mind over Matter: Reappraising Arousal Improves Cardiovascular and Cognitive Responses to Stress." *Journal of Experimental Psychology: General* 141, no. 3 (2012): 417–22. See also: Jamieson, Jeremy P., Matthew K. Nock, and Wendy Berry Mendes. "Changing the Conceptualization of Stress in Social Anxiety Disorder Affective and Physiological Consequences." *Clinical Psychological Science* 1, no. 4 (2013): 363–74.

Jamieson hired observers to analyze . . . Beltzer, Miranda L., Matthew K. Nock, Brett J. Peters, and Jeremy P. Jamieson. "Rethinking Butterflies: The Affective, Physiological, and Performance Effects of Reappraising Arousal During Social Evaluation." *Emotion* 14, no. 4 (2014): 761–68.

In Jamieson's study, and in many . . . Mauss, Iris, Frank Wilhelm, and James Gross. "Is There Less to Social Anxiety Than Meets the Eye? Emotion Experience, Expression, and Bodily Responding." *Cognition and Emotion* 18, no. 5 (2004): 631–42. See also Anderson, Emily R., and Debra A. Hope. "The Relationship Among Social Phobia, Objective and Perceived Physiological Reactivity, and Anxiety Sensitivity in an Adolescent Population." *Journal of Anxiety Disorders* 23, no. 1 (2009): 18–26.

Sue Cotter recently retired . . . Personal interview conducted with Sue Cotter on December 4, 2014.

In this study, a team of . . . Lambert, Jessica E., Charles C. Benight, Tamra Wong, and Lesley E. Johnson. "Cognitive Bias in the Interpretation of Physiological Sensations, Coping Self-Efficacy, and Psychological Distress After Intimate Partner Violence." *Psychological Trauma: Theory, Research, Practice, and Policy* 5, no. 5 (2013): 494–500.

Knowing that you are adequate . . . Benight, Charles C., and Albert Bandura. "Social Cognitive Theory of Posttraumatic Recovery: The Role of Perceived Self-Efficacy." *Behaviour Research and Therapy* 42, no. 10 (2004): 1129–48.

Chapter 5. Connect: How Caring Creates Resilience

Looking at both animal . . . Taylor, Shelley E., Laura Cousino Klein, Brian P. Lewis, Tara L. Gruenewald, Regan A.R. Gurung, and John A. Updegraff. "Biobehavioral Responses to Stress in Females: Tend-and-Befriend, Not Fight-or-Flight." *Psychological Review* 107, no. 3 (2000): 411–29. Taylor, Shelley E., and Sarah L. Master. "Social Responses to Stress: The Tend-and-Befriend Model." In *The Handbook of Stress Science: Biology, Psychology, and Health*, edited by Richard Contrada and Andrew Baum, 101–9. New York: Spinger, 2011.

It can also unleash . . . Geary, David C., and Mark V. Flinn. "Sex Differences in Behavioral and Hormonal Response to Social Threat: Commentary on Taylor et al. (2000)." Psychological Review 104, no. 4 (2002): 745–50. Buchanan, Tony W., and Stephanie D. Preston. "Stress Leads to Prosocial Action in Immediate Need Situations." *Frontiers in Behavioral Neuroscience* 8, no. 5 (2014): 1–6.

Koranyi, Nicolas, and Klaus Rothermund. "Automatic Coping Mechanisms in Committed Relationships: Increased Interpersonal Trust as a Response to Stress." *Journal of Experimental Social Psychology* 48, no. 1 (2012): 180–85.

But this is just one part . . . Keltner, Dacher, Aleksandr Kogan, Paul K. Piff, and Sarina R. Saturn. "The Sociocultural Appraisals, Values, and Emotions (SAVE) Framework of Prosociality: Core Processes from Gene to Meme." *Annual Review of Psychology* 65 (2014): 425–60.

A study by neuroscientists at UCLA . . . Inagaki, Tristen K., and Naomi I. Eisenberger. "Neural Correlates of Giving Support to a Loved One." *Psychosomatic Medicine* 74, no. 1 (2012): 3–7.

Time scarcity is not just a stressful . . . Strazdins, Lyndall, Amy L. Griffin, Dorothy H. Broom, Cathy Banwell, Rosemary Korda, Jane Dixon, Francesco Paolucci, and John Glover. "Time Scarcity: Another Health Inequality?" *Environment and Planning, Part A* 43, no. 3 (2011): 545–59.

The Wharton researchers summarized . . . Mogilner, Cassie, Zoë Chance, and Michael I. Norton. "Giving Time Gives You Time." *Psychological Science* 23, no. 10 (2012): 1233–38.

For example, people wrongly predict . . . Aknin, Lara B., Elizabeth W. Dunn, and Michael I. Norton. "Happiness Runs in a Circular Motion: Evidence for a Positive Feedback Loop Between Prosocial Spending and Happiness." *Journal of Happiness Studies* 13, no. 2 (2012): 347–55.

The brain changes were stronger . . . Harbaugh, William T., Ulrich Mayr, and Daniel R. Burghart. "Neural Responses to Taxation and Voluntary Giving Reveal Motives for Charitable Donations." *Science* 316, no. 5831 (2007): 1622–25.

Jennifer Crocker was on a sabbatical . . . Personal interview conducted with Jennifer Crocker on April 29, 2014.

The workshop focused on the costs . . . I have not taken the notes

Learning as Leadership workshop that inspired Jennifer Crocker's research, but you can learn more about their programs at www.learnaslead.com.

It is more about how . . . Nuer, Lara. "Learning as Leadership: A Methodology for Organizational Change Through Personal Mastery." Performance Improvement 38, no. 10 (1999): 9–13.

Crocker and her colleagues . . . Crocker, Jennifer, Marc-Andre Olivier, and Noah Nuer. "Self-Image Goals and Compassionate Goals: Costs and Benefits." *Self and Identity* 8, no. 2–3 (2009): 251–69. Crocker, Jennifer. "The Paradoxical Consequences of Interpersonal Goals: Relationships, Distress, and the Self." *Psychological Studies* 56, no. 1 (2011): 142–50. Crocker, Jennifer, Amy Canevello, and M. Liu. "Five Consequences of Self-Image and Compassionate Goals." *Advances in Experimental Social Psychology* 45 (2012): 229–77.

In one study, Crocker and her . . . Abelson, James L., Thane M. Erickson, Stefanie E. Mayer, Jennifer Crocker, Hedieh Briggs, Nestor L. Lopez-Duran, and Israel Liberzon. "Brief Cognitive Intervention Can Modulate Neuroendocrine Stress Responses to the Trier Social Stress Test: Buffering Effects of a Compassionate Goal Orientation." *Psychoneuroendocrinology* 44 (2014): 60–70.

David Yeager, whom we met . . . Yeager, David S., Marlone Henderson, David Paunesku, Gregory M. Walton, Sidney D'Mello, Brian J. Spitzer, and Angela Lee Duckworth. "Boring but Important: A Self-Transcendent Purpose for Learning Fosters Academic Self-Regulation." *Regulation* (2014, in press).

It also increased activity . . . Jack, Anthony I., Richard E. Boyatzis, Masud S. Khawaja, Angela M. Passarelli, and Regina L. Leckie. "Visioning in the Brain: An fMRI Study of Inspirational Coaching and Mentoring." *Social Neuroscience* 8, no. 4 (2013): 369–84.

Monica Worline is a founding member . . . Personal interview conducted with Monica Worline on August 5, 2014.

254

In 2013, researchers at . . . Hernandez, Morela, Megan F. Hess, and Jared D. Harris. "Leaning into the Wind: Hardship, Stakeholder Relationships, and Organizational Resilience." In *Academy of Management Proceedings*, vol. 2013, no. 1, 16640. Academy of Management, 2013.

They spend more time caring . . . Frazier, Patricia, Christiaan Greer, Susanne Gabrielsen, Howard Tennen, Crystal Park, and Patricia Tomich. "The Relation Between Trauma Exposure and Prosocial Behavior." *Psychological Trauma: Theory, Research, Practice, and Policy* 5, no. 3 (2013): 286–94.

As a researcher, he had intended . . . Staub, Ervin, and Johanna Vollhardt. "Altruism Born of Suffering: The Roots of Caring and Helping After Victimization and Other Trauma." *American Journal of Orthopsychiatry* 78, no. 3 (2008): 267–80.

More broadly, Staub has found . . . Vollhardt, Johanna R., and Ervin Staub. "Inclusive Altruism Born of Suffering: The Relationship Between Adversity and Prosocial Attitudes and Behavior Toward Disadvantaged Outgroups." *American Journal of Orthopsychiatry* 81, no. 3 (2011): 307–15.

In other words, when you think . . . Taylor, Peter James, Patricia Gooding, Alex M. Wood, and Nicholas Tarrier. "The Role of Defeat and Entrapment in Depression, Anxiety, and Suicide." *Psychological Bulletin* 137, no. 3 (2011): 391–420.

As one woman who served food . . . Steffen, Seana Lowe, and Alice Fothergill. "9/11 Volunteerism: A Pathway to Personal Healing and Community Engagement." *Social Science Journal* 46, no. 1 (2009): 29–46.

People who volunteer after . . . Cristea, Ioana A., Emanuele Legge, Marta Prosperi, Mario Guazzelli, Daniel David, and Claudio Gentili. "Moderating Effects of Empathic Concern and Personal Distress on the Emotional Reactions of Disaster Volunteers." *Disasters* 38, no. 4 (2014): 740–52.

After the death of a spouse . . . Brown, Stephanie L., R. Michael Brown, James S. House, and Dylan M. Smith. "Coping with Spousal Loss: Potential Buffering Effects of Self-Reported Helping Behavior." *Personality and Social Psychology Bulletin* 34, no. 6 (2008): 849–61.

Survivors of a natural disaster . . . Doran, Jennifer M., Ani Kalayjian, Loren Toussaint, and Diana Maria Mendez. "Posttraumatic Stress and Meaning Making in Mexico City." *Psychology and Developing Societies* 26, no. 1 (2014): 91–114.

Among people living with . . . Arnstein, Paul, Michelle Vidal, Carol Wells-Federman, Betty Morgan, and Margaret Caudill. "From Chronic Pain Patient to Peer: Benefits and Risks of Volunteering." *Pain Management Nursing* 3, no. 3 (2002): 94–103.

Victims of a terrorist attack . . . Kleinman, Stuart B. "A Terrorist Hijacking: Victims' Experiences Initially and 9 Years Later." *Journal of Traumatic Stress* 2, no. 1 (1989): 49–58.

After enduring a life-threatening . . . Sullivan, Gwynn B., and Martin J. Sullivan. "Promoting Wellness in Cardiac Rehabilitation: Exploring the Role of Altruism." *Journal of Cardiovascular Nursing* 11, no. 3 (1997): 43–52.

In one groundbreaking study . . . Poulin, Michael J., and E. Alison Holman. "Helping Hands, Healthy Body? Oxytocin Receptor Gene and Prosocial Behavior Interact to Buffer the Association Between Stress and Physical Health." *Hormones and Behavior* 63, no. 3 (2013): 510–17.

The researchers tracked 846 men . . . Poulin, Michael J., Stephanie L. Brown, Amanda J. Dillard, and Dylan M. Smith. "Giving to Others and the Association Between Stress and Mortality." *American Journal of Public Health* 103, no. 9 (2013): 1649–55.

A study at the University at Buffalo . . . Poulin, Michael J., and E. Alison Holman. "Helping Hands, Healthy Body? Oxytocin Receptor Gene and Prosocial Behavior Interact to Buffer the Association between Stress and Physical Health." *Hormones and Behavior* 63, no. 3 (2013): 510–17.

"The same young adults . . ." Quotes from EMS Corps trainees and Alameda County Health Care Services Agency director Alex Briscoe appear in these videos, produced by EMS Corps: Emergency Medical Services Corps (EMS Corps): "Providing an Opportunity for Young Men to Become Competent and Successful Health Care Providers" (http://www.rwjf.org/en/about-rwjf/newsroom /newsroom-content/2014/01/ems-corps-video.html) and "EMS Corps Students Reflect on Heart 2 Heart Door-to-Door Blood Pressure Screening Event (https://www.youtube.com/watch?v= gSkwqLqP2tE).

In one study, students . . . Schreier, Hannah M.C., Kimberly A. Schonert-Reichl, and Edith Chen. "Effect of Volunteering on Risk Factors for Cardiovascular Disease in Adolescents: A Randomized Controlled Trial." *JAMA Pediatrics* 167, no. 4 (2013): 327–32.

The veterans who participate . . . Yount, Rick, Elspeth Cameron Ritchie, Matthew St. Laurent, Perry Chumley, and Meg Daley Olmert. "The Role of Service Dog Training in the Treatment of Combat-Related PTSD." *Psychiatric Annals* 43, no. 6 (2013): 292–95.

"I held his hand and said a prayer . . ." Direct quote from an inmate caregiver about his experience caring for a dying inmate. From Loeb, Susan J., Christopher S. Hollenbeak, Janice Penrod, Carol A. Smith, Erin Kitt-Lewis, and Sarah B. Crouse. "Care and Companionship in an Isolating Environment: Inmates Attending to Dying Peers." *Journal of Forensic Nursing* 9, no. 1 (2013): 35–44. The quote is on page 39.

Penn State's Loeb has . . . Ibid. See also Wright, Kevin N., and Laura Bronstein. "An Organizational Analysis of Prison Hospice." *Prison Journal* 87, no. 4 (2007): 391–407.

As one wrote in an anonymous survey . . . Cloyes, Kristin G., Susan J. Rosenkranz, Dawn Wold, Patricia H. Berry, and Katherine P. Supiano. "To Be Truly Alive: Motivation Among Prison Inmate Hospice Volunteers and the Transformative Process of End-of-Life Peer Care Service." *American Journal of Hospice and Palliative Medicine* (2013): 1–14.

When inmate hospice volunteers . . . Ibid.

Look at the four statements below . . . These items are from the isolation and common humanity subscales of Kristin Neff's Self-Compassion Scale. Neff, Kristin D. "The Development and Validation of a Scale to Measure Self-Compassion." *Self and Identity* 2, no. 3 (2003): 223–50.

People who feel alone . . . Allen, Ashley Batts, and Mark R. Leary. "Self-Compassion, Stress, and Coping." *Social and Personality Psychology Compass* 4, no. 2 (2010): 107–118. Neff, Kristin D. "The Development and Validation of a Scale to Measure Self-Compassion." *Self and Identity* 2, no. 3 (2003): 223–50.

They are more open about . . . Gilbert, Paul, Kristen McEwan, Francisco Catarino, and Rita Baião. "Fears of Compassion in a Depressed Population Implication for Psychotherapy." *Journal of Depression and Anxiety S* 2 (2014): doi: 10.4172/2167-1044.S2-003. Jazaieri, Hooria, Geshe Thupten Jinpa, Kelly McGonigal, Erika L. Rosenberg, Joel Finkelstein, Emiliana Simon-Thomas, Margaret Cullen, James R. Doty, James J. Gross, and Philippe R. Goldin. "Enhancing Compassion: A Randomized Controlled Trial of a Compassion Cultivation Training Program." *Journal of Happiness Studies* 14, no. 4 (2013): 1113–26.

They are also more likely . . . Barnard, Laura K., and John F. Curry. "The Relationship of Clergy Burnout to Self-Compassion and Other Personality Dimensions." *Pastoral Psychology* 61, no. 2 (2012): 149–63. Raab, Kelley. "Mindfulness, Self-Compassion, and Empathy Among Health Care Professionals: A Review of the

Literature." *Journal of Health Care Chaplaincy* 20, no. 3 (2014): 95–108. Abaci, Ramazan, and Devrim Arda. "Relationship Between Self-Compassion and Job Satisfaction in White Collar Workers." *Procedia—Social and Behavioral Sciences* 106 (2013): 2241–47.

And yet, despite the benefits . . . Jordan, Alexander H., Benoît Monin, Carol S. Dweck, Benjamin J. Lovett, Oliver P. John, and James J. Gross. "Misery Has More Company Than People Think: Underestimating the Prevalence of Others' Negative Emotions." *Personality and Social Psychology Bulletin* 37, no. 1 (2011): 120–35.

"We often judge our insides . . ." Orsillo, Susan M., and Lizabeth Roemer. *The Mindful Way through Anxiety: Break Free from Chronic Worry and Reclaim Your Life* 161, Guilford Press, 2011.

Because the suffering of others . . . McGonigal, Kelly. "The Mindful Way to Self-Compassion." *Shambala Sun* (July 2011): 77.

Even though most people are aware . . . Fay, Adam J., Alexander H. Jordan, and Joyce Ehrlinger. "How Social Norms Promote Misleading Social Feedback and Inaccurate Self-Assessment." *Social and Personality Psychology Compass* 6, no. 2 (2012): 206–16.

Studies show that spending time . . . Burke, Moira, Cameron Marlow, and Thomas Lento. "Social Network Activity and Social Well-Being." In *Proceedings of the SIGCHI Conference on Human Factors in Computing Systems*, 1909–12. Association for Computing Machinery, 2010. Lou, Lai Lei, Zheng Yan, Amanda Nickerson, and Robert McMorris. "An Examination of the Reciprocal Relationship of Loneliness and Facebook Use Among First-Year College Students." *Journal of Educational Computing Research* 46, no. 1 (2012): 105–117. Krasnova, Hanna, Helena Wenninger, Thomas Widjaja, and Peter Buxmann. "Envy on Facebook: A Hidden Threat to Users' Life Satisfaction?" (2013).

This is a question I've explored . . . For more information about my research with the Stanford Center for Compassion and Altruism Research and Education (ccare.stanford.edu) on cultivating a mindset of common humanity, see Jazaieri, Hooria, Kelly McGonigal, Thupten Jinpa, James R. Doty, James J. Gross, and Philippe R. Goldin. "A Randomized Controlled Trial of Compassion Cultivation Training: Effects on Mindfulness, Affect, and Emotion Regulation." *Motivation and Emotion* 38, no. 1 (2014): 23–35. Jazaieri, Hooria, Geshe Thupten Jinpa, Kelly McGonigal, Erika L. Rosenberg, Joel Finkelstein, Emiliana Simon-Thomas, Margaret Cullen, James R. Doty, James J. Gross, and Philippe R. Goldin. "Enhancing Compassion: A Randomized Controlled Trial of a Compassion Cultivation Training Program." *Journal of Happiness Studies* 14, no. 4 (2013): 1113–26.

Flowers and Fernandez cofounded the Dinner Party . . . Information about the Dinner Party can be found at http://thedinnerparty.org/. Personal interview conducted with Lennon Flowers on August 18, 2014.

Like Flowers, who cofounded the Dinner Party . . . Garcia, Julie A., and Jennifer Crocker. "Reasons for Disclosing Depression Matter: The Consequences of Having Egosystem and Ecosystem Goals." *Social Science and Medicine* 67, no. 3 (2008): 453–62. Newheiser, Anna-Kaisa, and Manuela Barreto. "Hidden Costs of Hiding Stigma: Ironic Interpersonal Consequences of Concealing a Stigmatized Identity in Social Interactions." *Journal of Experimental Social Psychology* 52 (2014): 58–70.

Sole Train is a running and mentoring program . . . More information about Sole Train can be found at http://www.trinityinspires.org/sole-train/. Personal interview conducted with Jessica Leffler on March 21, 2014.

A student had brought in . . . Martha Ross, "Stress: It's Contagious," San Jose Mercury News, July 27, 2014, D1–D3.

A sympathetic stress response . . . Buchanan, Tony W., Sara L.

Bagley, R. Brent Stansfield, and Stephanie D. Preston. "The Empathic, Physiological Resonance of Stress." *Social Neuroscience* 7, no. 2 (2012): 191–201.

Chapter 6. Grow: How Adversity Makes You Stronger

For example, when people are asked . . . Aldwin, Carolyn M., Karen J. Sutton, and Margie Lachman. "The Development of Coping Resources in Adulthood." *Journal of Personality* 64, no. 4 (1996): 837–71.

Adversity, he claimed . . . Seery, Mark D., E. Alison Holman, and Roxane Cohen Silver. "Whatever Does Not Kill Us: Cumulative Lifetime Adversity, Vulnerability, and Resilience." *Journal of Personality and Social Psychology* 99, no. 6 (2010): 1025–41. Seery, Mark D. "Resilience a Silver Lining to Experiencing Adverse Life Events?" *Current Directions in Psychological Science* 20, no. 6 (2011): 390–94. Seery, Mark D., Raphael J. Leo, Shannon P. Lupien, Cheryl L. Kondrak, and Jessica L. Almonte. "An Upside to Adversity? Moderate Cumulative Lifetime Adversity Is Associated with Resilient Responses in the Face of Controlled Stressors." *Psychological Science* 24, no. 7 (2013): 1181–89. All quotes, along with some study details and interpretation, come from a personal conversation with Mark Seery on July 9, 2014.

Among adults with chronic back pain . . . Seery, Mark D., Raphael J. Leo, E. Alison Holman, and Roxane Cohen Silver. "Lifetime Exposure to Adversity Predicts Functional Impairment and Healthcare Utilization Among Individuals with Chronic Back Pain." *Pain* 150, no. 3 (2010): 507–15.

Police officers who have experienced . . . Burke, Karena J., and Jane Shakespeare-Finch. "Markers of Resilience in New Police Officers Appraisal of Potentially Traumatizing Events." *Traumatology* 17, no. 4 (2011): 52–60.

Thirteen first-generation college students . . . For more information about ScholarMatch, visit scholarmatch.org.

Because of this, their grades improved . . . Yeager, David Scott, Valerie Purdie-Vaughns, Julio Garcia, Nancy Apfel, Patti Brzustoski, Allison Master, William T. Hessert, Matthew E. Williams, and Geoffrey L. Cohen. "Breaking the Cycle of Mistrust: Wise Interventions to Provide Critical Feedback Across The Racial Divide." *Journal of Experimental Psychology: General* 143, no. 2 (2014): 804–24.

A coping style called shift-and-persist . . . Chen, Edith, and Gregory E. Miller. "Shift-and-Persist Strategies: Why Low Socioeconomic Status Isn't Always Bad for Health." *Perspectives on Psychological Science* 7, no. 2 (2012): 135–158.

Psychologists call this phenomenon *post-traumatic growth* . . . Tedeschi, Richard G., and Lawrence G. Calhoun. "Posttraumatic Growth: Conceptual Foundations and Empirical Evidence." *Psychological Inquiry* 15, no. 1 (2004): 1–18. Sample post-traumatic growth items from Tedeschi, Richard G., and Lawrence G. Calhoun. "The Posttraumatic Growth Inventory: Measuring the Positive Legacy of Trauma." *Journal of Traumatic Stress* 9, no. 3 (1996): 455–71.

However, it is far from unusual . . . Laufer, Avital, and Zahava Solomon. "Posttraumatic Symptoms and Posttraumatic Growth Among Israeli Youth Exposed to Terror Incidents." *Journal of Social and Clinical Psychology* 25, no. 4 (2006): 429–47. Siegel, Karolynn, and Eric W. Schrimshaw. "Perceiving Benefits in Adversity: Stress-Related Growth in Women Living with HIV/AIDS." *Social Science and Medicine* 51, no. 10 (2000): 1543–54. Shakespeare-Finch, Jane E., S.G. Smith, Kathryn M. Gow, Gary Embelton, and L. Baird. "The Prevalence of Post-Traumatic Growth in Emergency Ambulance Personnel." *Traumatology* 9, no. 1 (2003): 58–71.

As one 2013 review of research . . . Cho, Dalnim, and Crystal L. Park. "Growth Following Trauma: Overview and Current Status." *Terapia Psicologica* 31, no. 1 (2013): 69–79.

In fact, people routinely report . . . Baker, Jennifer M., Caroline Kelly, Lawrence G. Calhoun, Arnie Cann, and Richard G. Tedeschi. "An Examination of Posttraumatic Growth and Posttraumatic Depreciation: Two Exploratory Studies." *Journal of Loss and Trauma* 13, no. 5 (2008): 450–65. Tsai, J., R. El-Gabalawy, W.H. Sledge, S.M. Southwick, and R.H. Pietrzak. "Post-Traumatic Growth Among Veterans in the USA: Results from the National Health and Resilience in Veterans Study." *Psychological Medicine*: 1–15.

A 2014 analysis of forty-two studies Shakespeare-Finch, Jane, and Janine Lurie-Beck. "A Meta-Analytic Clarification of the Relationship Between Posttraumatic Growth and Symptoms of Posttraumatic Distress Disorder." *Journal of Anxiety Disorders* 28, no. 2 (2014): 223–29.

It ignites a psychological process . . . Kehl, Doris, Daniela Knuth, Markéta Holubová, Lynn Hulse, and Silke Schmidt. "Relationships Between Firefighters' Postevent Distress and Growth at Different Times After Distressing Incidents." *Traumatology* 20, no. 4 (2014): 253–61. Lowe, Sarah R., Emily E. Manove, and Jean E. Rhodes. "Posttraumatic Stress and Posttraumatic Growth Among Low-Income Mothers Who Survived Hurricane Katrina." *Journal of Consulting and Clinical Psychology* 81, no. 5 (2013): 877–89.

This was the case for Jennifer White . . . Information about Jennifer White's Hope After Project, including her personal story and how to get involved, is available at http://www.hopeafterproject.com. Personal interview conducted on December 12, 2014.

Men who find an upside . . . Affleck, Glenn, Howard Tennen, Sydney Croog, and Sol Levine. "Causal Attribution, Perceived Benefits, and Morbidity After a Heart Attack: An 8-Year Study." *Journal of Consulting and Clinical Psychology* 55, no. 1 (1987): 29–35.

HIV-positive women who recognize . . . Ickovics, Jeannette R., Stephanie Milan, Robert Boland, Ellie Schoenbaum, Paula Schuman, David Vlahov, and HIV Epidemiology Research Study (HERS) Group. "Psychological Resources Protect Health: 5-Year Survival and Immune Function Among HIV-Infected Women from Four U.S. Cities." *AIDS* 20, no. 14 (2006): 1851–60.

Among men and women . . . Danoff-Burg, Sharon, and Tracey A. Revenson. "Benefit-Finding Among Patients with Rheumatoid Arthritis: Positive Effects on Interpersonal Relationships." *Journal of Behavioral Medicine* 28, no. 1 (2005): 91–103.

For instance, caregivers who find . . . Mavandadi, Shahrzad, Roseanne Dobkin, Eugenia Mamikonyan, Steven Sayers, Thomas Ten Have, and Daniel Weintraub. "Benefit Finding and Relationship Quality in Parkinson's Disease: A Pilot Dyadic Analysis of Husbands and Wives." *Journal of Family Psychology* 28, no. 5 (2014): 728–34.

In teens with diabetes . . . Tran, Vincent, Deborah J. Wiebe, Katherine T. Fortenberry, Jorie M. Butler, and Cynthia A. Berg. "Benefit Finding, Affective Reactions to Diabetes Stress, and Diabetes Management Among Early Adolescents." *Health Psychology* 30, no. 2 (2011): 212–19.

The protective effect is strongest . . . Wood, Michael D., Thomas W. Britt, Jeffrey L. Thomas, Robert P. Klocko, and Paul D. Bliese. "Buffering Effects of Benefit Finding in a War Environment." *Military Psychology* 23, no. 2 (2011): 202–19.

People who find benefit in . . . Cassidy, Tony, Marian McLaughlin, and Melanie Giles. "Benefit Finding in Response to General Life Stress: Measurement and Correlates." *Health Psychology and Behavioral Medicine* 2, no. 1 (2014): 268–82.

They then are more likely . . . Pakenham, Kenneth I., Kate Sofronoff, and Christina Samios. "Finding Meaning in Parenting a Child with Asperger Syndrome: Correlates of Sense Making and Benefit Finding." *Research in Developmental Disabilities* 25, no. 3 (2004): 245–64.

In the laboratory, people who . . . Bower, Julienne E., Carissa A. Low, Judith Tedlie Moskowitz, Saviz Sepah, and Elissa Epel. "Benefit Finding and Physical Health: Positive Psychological Changes and Enhanced Allostasis." *Social and Personality Psychology Compass* 2, no. 1 (2008): 223–44. Bower, Julienne E., Judith Tedlie Moskowitz, and Elissa Epel. "Is Benefit Finding Good for Your Health? Pathways Linking Positive Life Changes After Stress and Physical Health Outcomes." *Current Directions in Psychological Science* 18, no. 6 (2009): 337–41.

For example, people who report both . . . Butler, Lisa D. "Growing Pains: Commentary on the Field Of Posttraumatic Growth and Hobfoll and Colleagues' Recent Contributions to It." *Applied Psychology* 56, no. 3 (2007): 367–78.

Survivors of a life-threatening disease . . . Cheng, Cecilia, Wai-man Wong, and Kenneth W. Tsang. "Perception of Benefits and Costs During SARS Outbreak: An 18-Month Prospective Study." *Journal of Consulting and Clinical Psychology* 74, no. 5 (2006): 870–79.

They also reported less desire . . . McCullough, Michael E., Lindsey M. Root, and Adam D. Cohen. "Writing About the Benefits of an Interpersonal Transgression Facilitates Forgiveness." *Journal of Consulting and Clinical Psychology* 74, no. 5 (2006): 887–97.

Amazingly, another study found . . . vanOyen Witvliet, Charlotte, Ross W. Knoll, Nova G. Hinman, and Paul A. DeYoung. "Compassion-Focused Reappraisal, Benefit-Focused Reappraisal, and Rumination After an Interpersonal Offense: Emotion-Regulation Implications for Subjective Emotion, Linguistic Responses, and Physiology." *Journal of Positive Psychology* 5, no. 3 (2010): 226–42.

Benefit-finding is associated . . . Rabe, Sirko, Tanja Zöllner, Andreas Maercker, and Anke Karl. "Neural Correlates of Posttraumatic Growth After Severe Motor Vehicle Accidents." *Journal of Consulting and Clinical Psychology* 74, no. 5 (2006): 880–86.

Those who struggled the most . . . Danoff-Burg, Sharon, John D. Agee, Norman R. Romanoff, Joel M. Kremer, and James M. Strosberg. "Benefit Finding and Expressive Writing in Adults with Lupus or Rheumatoid Arthritis." *Psychology and Health* 21, no. 5 (2006): 651–65.

Tellingly, women who had been . . . Stanton, Annette L., Sharon Danoff-Burg, Lisa A. Sworowski, Charlotte A. Collins, Ann D. Branstetter, Alicia Rodriguez-Hanley, Sarah B. Kirk, and Jennifer L. Austenfeld. "Randomized, Controlled Trial of Written Emotional Expression and Benefit Finding in Breast Cancer Patients." *Journal of Clinical Oncology* 20, no. 20 (2002): 4160–68.

Another intervention asked those caring . . . Cheng, Sheung-Tak, Rosanna W.L. Lau, Emily P.M. Mak, Natalie S.S. Ng, and Linda C.W. Lam. "Benefit-Finding Intervention for Alzheimer Caregivers: Conceptual Framework, Implementation Issues, and Preliminary Efficacy." *Gerontologist* 54, no. 6 (2014): 1049–58.

The article Wiltenburg wrote . . . Wiltenburg, Mary. "She Doesn't Want to Share Her Grief with a Nation." *Christian Science Monitor.* September 3, 2002. Wiltenburg, Mary. "9/11 Hijacking Victim's Family Expanded, Even Without Him." *Christian Science Monitor.* September 9, 2011. Personal interview conducted with Mary Wiltenburg on September 16, 2014.

One shocking study found that . . . Holman, E. Alison, Dana Rose Garfin, and Roxane Cohen Silver. "Media's Role in Broadcasting Acute Stress Following the Boston Marathon Bombings." *Proceedings of the National Academy of Sciences* 111, no. 1 (2014): 93–98. Pfefferbaum, Betty, Elana Newman, Summer D. Nelson, Pascal Nitiéma, Rose L. Pfefferbaum, and Ambreen Rahman. "Disaster

Media Coverage and Psychological Outcomes: Descriptive Findings in the Extant Research." *Current Psychiatry Reports* 16, no. 9 (2014): 1–7.

A 2014 study of U.S. adults . . . "The GfK Group Project Report for the National Survey of Fears" (2014). Available at http://www.chapman.edu/wilkinson/research-centers/babbie-center/survey-american-fears.aspx.

Findings like this motivate Images and Voices of Hope (IVOH) . . . More information about IVOH can be found at http://ivoh.org/. Personal interview conducted with Mallory Jean Tenore on February 12, 2014.

Vicarious growth was most commonly . . . Arnold, Debora, Lawrence G. Calhoun, Richard Tedeschi, and Arnie Cann. "Vicarious Posttraumatic Growth in Psychotherapy." *Journal of Humanistic Psychology* 45, no. 2 (2005): 239–63. Barrington, Allysa, and Jane E. Shakespeare-Finch. "Giving Voice to Service Providers Who Work with Survivors of Torture and Trauma." *Qualitative Health Research* 24, no. 12 (2014). 1686–99. Hernández, Pilar, David Gangsei, and David Engstrom. "Vicarious Resilience: A New Concept in Work With Those Who Survive Trauma." *Family Process* 46, no. 2 (2007): 229–41. Acevedo, Victoria Eugenia, and Pilar Hernandez-Wolfe. "Vicarious Resilience: An Exploration of Teachers and Children's Resilience in Highly Challenging Social Contexts." *Journal of Aggression, Maltreatment, and Trauma* 23, no. 5 (2014): 473–93. Inocencio Soares, Nataly Tsumura, and Mauren Teresa Grubisich Mendes Tacla. "Experience of Nursing Staff Facing the Hospitalization of Burned Children." *Investigación y Educación en Enfermería* 32, no. 1 (2014): 49–59.

The participants reported not only . . . Abel, Lisa, Casie Walker, Christina Samios, and Larissa Morozow. "Vicarious Posttraumatic

Growth: Predictors of Growth and Relationships with Adjustment." *Traumatology* 20, no. 1 (2014): 9–18.

The process of learning and . . . Tosone, Carol, Jennifer Bauwens, and Marc Glassman. "The Shared Traumatic and Professional Posttraumatic Growth Inventory." *Research on Social Work Practice* (ahead of print, 2014). doi: 10.1177/1049731514549814.

We often think about . . . Therapist's quote taken from Engstrom, David, Pilar Hernandez, and David Gangsei. "Vicarious Resilience: A Qualitative Investigation into Its Description." *Traumatology* 14, no. 3 (2008): 13–21.

Six months after recruits . . . Shochet, Ian M., Jane Shakespeare-Finch, Cameron Craig, Colette Roos, Astrid Wurfl, Rebecca Hoge, Ross McD Young, and Paula Brough. "The Development and Implementation of the Promoting Resilient Officers (PRO) Program." *Traumatology* 17, no. 4 (2011): 43–51. Shakespeare-Finch, Jane E., Ian M. Shochet, Colette R. Roos, Cameron Craig, Deanne Armstrong, Ross McD Young, and Astrid Wurfl. "Promoting Posttraumatic Growth in Police Recruits: Preliminary Results of a Randomised Controlled Resilience Intervention Trial." In *Australian and New Zealand Disaster and Emergency Management Conference*, Association for Sustainability in Business, QT Gold Coast Hotel, Surfers Paradise (2014).

These outcomes don't seem . . . Hayes, Steven C., Jason B. Luoma, Frank W. Bond, Akihiko Masuda, and Jason Lillis. "Acceptance and Commitment Therapy: Model, Processes and Outcomes." *Behaviour Research and Therapy* 44, no. 1 (2006): 1–25. See also Bond, Frank W., Steven C. Hayes, Ruth A. Baer, Kenneth M. Carpenter, Nigel Guenole, Holly K. Orcutt, Tom Waltz, and Robert D. Zettle. "Preliminary Psychometric Properties of the Acceptance and Action Questionnaire—II: A Revised Measure of Psychological Inflexibility and Experiential Avoidance." *Behavior Therapy* 42, no. 4 (2011): 676–88.

index

Page numbers in **bold** indicate tables.

ALSO BY KELLY McGONIGAL, Ph.D.

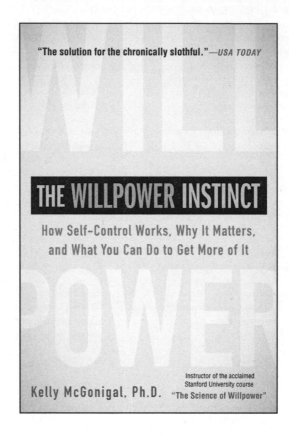

The Willpower Instinct is the first book to explain the new science of self-control and how it can be harnessed to improve our health, happiness, and productivity.